MAKE AN
IMPACT

The Six Habits of Highly Influential People

FAB GIOVANETTI

hey,

Welcome to this wonderful book brought to you by That Guy's House Publishing.

At That Guy's House we believe in real and raw wellness books that inspire the reader from a place of authenticity and honesty.

This book has been carefully crafted by both the author and publisher with the intention that it will bring you a glimmer of hope, a rush of inspiration and sensation of inner peace.

It is our hope that you thoroughly enjoy this book and pass it onto friends who may also be in need of a glimpse into their own magnificence.

Have a wonderful day.

Love,

Sean Patrick

That Guy.

To Matteo

"I mean, they say you die twice. One time when you stop breathing and a second time, a bit later on, when somebody says your name for the last time."

-BANKSY

Table of Content

PART ONE:
INTRODUCTION

Foreword by Lauren Armes

It's unthinkable really, upon reflection… to insist that somebody who is fasting accompany you to the Selfridges Food Hall. Which is exactly what I did to Fab the first time we met in London's West End. But Fab, in the truly gracious and generous manner for which I have come to appreciate her, relented willingly, chewing my ear off the whole way along Oxford Street, dodging the peak hour crowds and semi-jogging to keep up with my long stride.

We weren't to know at the time, 4 years ago, that the wellness industry would evolve in quite the way (or at the speed) it has. Nor were we to know that the concept of influence would become so prevalent and that, as a consequence, this book would be quite so needed. With Fab, however, I sensed from day one an inherent knowing that a growing community of people needed support to fully understand the power of their own message.

She has, through sheer determination, a willingness to listen, respond, and ultimately deliver, built a community bound by a shared passion for a cause. Fab is, in her own right, a leader and a pioneer – something garnered only by an individual respected by their followers. It takes this experience in building influence, to write meaningfully about it.

Influence, by its very nature, requires that we be known to others. We become known because of who we are, who we're becoming, and what we represent to those around us. The mechanisms by which we can achieve a certain status in society, are no longer bound by geography or culture... as introverts, minorities and pseudo-experts step up onto the world stage. But more and more it seems that authenticity is also a prerequisite; an attribute that those who influence must give concerted effort to cultivating. An attribute, I'll add, which is truly embodied by Fab Giovanetti.

If it weren't for influence, my business simply would not exist. And yet for the first 2 years of building Welltodo I refrained from so much as mentioning my own name on the company website. There was no 'about us' page to be found. Because, the truth is, technology and the transparency it provides, is adding new layers to the concept of influence day by day. As a result, we feel more at risk of being exposed or 'found out'. It's a conflict between the desire to speak up about what we believe whilst fearing the judgement of those who disagree.

Despite this conflict, there has never been a more important time for both budding and established entrepreneurs to think about how to garner, and why, influence is so critical. It takes a considerably depth of insight, experience and enquiry to fully understand the long standing impact of influence on our culture, our businesses and our ability to build authentic identities for ourselves. It's a necessary insight which this book so generously provides.

Marianne Williamson said it herself, that we are not frightened by our darkness, but rather our light and power. That is, who we have the potential to be in the world and the influence with which we are able to live and lead.

The problem for most of us, is that we are afraid of everything that comes with power and influence, and the blueprint is usually a negative one. For example, we fear that power and influence will mean expectation, criticism, pressure to be more or less. We fear the responsibility that comes with power, and not just because Spiderman says that it does.

In her debut book, Fab asks us to look beyond the definition of influence that has been prescribed by social media, and consider the inherent desire of us all to have an impact, leave a lasting legacy, and to learn from those that we admire – to influence and be influenced. And in an age where 'influencer' is a legitimate job title, you're picking up this book at the right time if you seek to truly understand what this role encompasses.

If you've ever wondered what your role is in this new generation of influencers, or how it can and will impact the commerciality of what you do (for work or play), then you're in the right place. Arming yourself with the practical applications of, and strategies with which to acquire real and lasting influence, will create vast opportunities and unlock enormous possibility in your life. In the pages that follow, you'll be taken by the hand and gently pulled in the direction of authentic power and intentional leadership – which is most certainly what the world needs more of right now.

Lauren Armes

Founder of Welltodo and Business Coach

As featured in Forbes, ES, Women's Health, Glamour, Red and Cosmopolitan

London, United Kingdom

Introduction

Well, my Dear Reader, let me tell you something from the get-go.

I am so excited. No seriously, I cannot believe you are here. I wish I could grab your gorgeous face and give you a big, fat kiss - on the cheek of course (come on, we just met).

This is set to be a stellar ride. I can feel it. You know that feeling of butterflies in the stomach?

That's exactly how I feel every time you open this book and read this introduction. Crazy how the fourth wall works, uh?

I am so humbled to have you here with me, and this is why I want to make a promise to you.

I promise to be 100% honest and transparent with you. Just like we were old time buddies. Somehow though, we are already buddies.

Our paths crossed because both of us know that the key to a happier, more fulfilling life is to be committed to leaving a positive mark on this Earth.

I still remember the time I watched that masterpiece that is *Into the Wild* (bawling my eyes out for probably a good half of it). I remember the quote *"happiness is real, only when it's shared"*.

That is it, right there.

How can you be happier if the only person you are trying to have an impact on is yourself?

What I did in this book is simple: I started doing what I do best.

I asked questions.

I investigated.

I extrapolated (and got lost in studies and research).

This all happened because I asked myself a very simple question, and let's be honest, that's precisely how all the best adventures begin.

A tale of a Crowdfunding Campaign

You know those moments you remember vividly? The ones that are stuck in your head, and you cannot shake off?

This is one of those.

I am coming back home from a few weeks visiting my family back in Italy. I am on a train from London to the outskirts. I am scrolling through my emails, trying to ignore the feelings that are bubbling deep down inside me. I can hear the noises around me, the muffled voices and the fast train sprinting to its next stop.

My forehead feels hot and sticky, and my eyes are burning.

I am going through a time of mourning, loss, and uncertainty. In this moment in time, my personal life is incredibly overwhelming, I have to start things all over again, and the business is plummeting into the abyss. My phone buzzes, and there it is: I receive an email I do not want to receive.

I stare at it, holding onto my suitcase; as the train stops, and I almost fall on it. I sigh, and I can feel my eyes burning under my sunglasses: I feel the tears falling down and tarnishing them.

I write a very simple message to my best friend. "I cannot do this anymore." I write. "I want out". She knows exactly what I mean. I do believe that soulmates do not need many words. They just know.

She calls me straight away: "Where are you? Are you alone?"

"I am on the train" I manage to say, before starting to cry uncontrollably "I cannot do this anymore" I keep murmuring.

I can hear her silently holding the space for me on the other end of the phone. After a few seconds, she is telling me all the right things - she has the ability to do that.

"Focus on what you can control", she says.

"You are not alone, and you know this. This is a safe space", she continues.

Fast-forward to a couple of days later, when I decided that I was going to set up a Crowdfunding page for the book you are currently holding.

I knew I had to do it, and deep inside me I knew I would fully fund it - apparently, only one out of five crowdfunding campaigns are fully supported. My campaign was about giving myself permission to be vulnerable. Ask people to believe in my vision and be part of it. To help me, help them.

As I sat on the floor of a 6.45pm train, on a hot early Summer day, I realised I was meant to do this. I was meant to be here, and I needed the people that I was serving every day to see it and feel it with me.

It's been a crazy ride: throughout my Crowdfunding adventure, I took the time to piece my life together, reassess my priorities and work harder than ever before to be of genuine service for my people.

I can tell I have never been prouder of you for picking up this book. Your support, your genuine love and passion mean the world. Without you, I would not be here today, my Dear Reader. You rock my world, and I genuinely hope you'll learn from this book as much as I did by writing it.

A History of

Influence

What is influence anyway?

I once heard this statement:

"Influence is leading, not trying to appease people by not saying the wrong thing".

"What if people are trying to get their message across, and by doing so, they have to compromise?" I answered in a heartbeat, trying to hide how defensive that made me feel.

Do we really have to, though?

As influencers, or people with considerable influence, do we really have to compromise our views and ideas? And what does being an influencer mean anyway?

Here's one explanation.

"(Marketing), a person or group that has the ability to influence the behaviour or opinion of others: the influencer is the individual whose effect on the purchase decision is in some way significant or authoritative" (Cambridge English Dictionary, 2018)

I am fortunate enough to know quite a few very influential people in my line of work, and I could even stretch to call myself one.

I work with people who want to grow their influence and make a positive change. And yet, some of us, instead of realising the incredible impact we may have on 100 people with just one picture, are still feeling discouraged when the number of people who we influence is not above one million!

When I started my quest, I set out to bring perspective to what, in my personal opinion, being an influencer is. Furthermore, after researching and cross-referencing the habits and beliefs of over 1,500 influencers, I set myself to define clearly what makes an *influencer.*

They always say you should write a book with one person in mind and as I am writing this, I realise I do not really have just one person in my head. Instead I have 10,500 people; those who I have touched in some way via our online community, the Health Bloggers Community. Members came, and members went, and some of them are off creating incredible things in the world (and I could not be more proud of each and every achievement that has come through the Health Bloggers Community).

No wonder my affectionate nickname is 'Mama Fab'.

I remember standing on a wooden box, in a local gym above a famous health food shop in South London, talking to over 30 people about what my humble group of bloggers was going to become. Looking back to that day, standing on that wooden box, I cannot help but ask myself this very simple question;

Am I an influencer? In fact, aren't we all, really?

I believe that most people who want to become a professional in the blogging industry (health and wellness) have a big responsibility when influencing others. It's not just about consumer choices or the perfect face mask. It's about making a positive impact, looking to inspire a change in people's behaviours and mindsets.

It transcends from within you and expands onto how you are going to impact others.

If we want to go down that route, I'd say as humans we are wired to create a legacy.

Whether it is the innate drive to become parents and give the gift of life, or create an incredible business (hell, even writing a book to some extent), we are wired to think outside ourselves and as you'll see by reading this book that this is something almost every influencer has in common.

I know what you must be wondering; can we really pinpoint common habits or traits that make some people more successful than others in harnessing their influence?

After extensive research, I do believe that the answer is "*Yes*". This is because these habits transcend our time.

You see, there is a transcendental difference between evergreen books and expendable books.

I do believe that, when you really find a pain point, or a specific set of traits and rules that are inherently linked with our psychology as humans, rather than marketing and business "how-to's", you create a timeless resource.

It does not matter whether you are on Instagram or influencing people by busking on the street, you can transfer each and every single habit to another industry or environment.

To prove my point, I was listening to Tim Ferris talk about his first book, *The Four Hour Work Week*. In an interview on his podcast[1] he pointed out that, by having a particular friend in mind trying to find a very specific solution to his problem, he created a book that transcends time. Some tools may become obsolete, but the core of the book and the actual strategies go beyond tools - and it's probably among my top 10 books to read.

This is why you are very unlikely to find a series of URLs jotted down in this book. The research I carried out was based on human behaviour, as well as studies from specific papers, articles, as well as books that go way beyond the current trends. It's very accurate in a way, as *influencer marketing* (as a buzzword) may be gone in 5 to 10 years' time. However, the idea is that influence exists at the core of who we are as humans, and taps into our emotion and behaviour.

The truth is straightforward, and also, a bit offensive - I hope you do not mind me being so blunt with you, right from this introduction.

As humans, we are inherently lazy.

Yes, influence can be linked to our inherent laziness, as we rely on influence because we don't have to figure things out for ourselves. But we also do it because of social pressure - an incredibly strong drive, now amplified with the advent of online influence.[2]

Should influencers lead, or should they compromise?

Born to influence, born to lead

Leadership is commonly defined as a social influence process even more than a trait: leaders are the ones who can determine a group's set of goals, assign tasks and challenges to reach those goals and influence the community and culture that will naturally start to develop.[3]

Influencers are, therefore, leaders. They lead by tapping into emotions that are at the core of our human nature.

Influence is at the core of who we are. It is the need for empathic connection, which shapes itself through the idea of emotional mimicry.

Let me lead with an example: when we see another person expressing an emotion, something as simple as a smile, cells in our brain, called mirror neurons, begin to fire, making us smile as well.

Leaders tap into our emotions, but leaders are also at the very core of what inspires us, and positively impacts our behaviour. It's interesting how plenty of books have been written about leadership, and still, someone has yet to see the correlation between influence and leadership as an emotional connection.

However, more and more, leadership books tend to explore behaviours of persuasion and programming. This proves my point exactly, my Dear Reader.

We could argue that, if you want to have an impact on people and become an expert influencer, you must be able to understand (and, I'd like to add, accept) the presence of psychological patterns and understand how everyday objects and surroundings shape and control our behaviour.

Influence is at the core of being human, nevertheless, harnessing our influence and channelling into inspiring a positive change is a conscious choice that requires habits to be developed.

If you are looking to grow, harness and refine your influence, then please do not stand in the doorway. Come on inside, I have freshly baked cookies, and some delicious coffee for you. All I ask is that you please leave your shoes in the hall.

Oh, and welcome home.

The History of influence

"Leadership is not about a title or a designation. It's about impact, influence and inspiration. Impact involves getting results, influence is about spreading the passion you have for your work, and you have to inspire teammates and customers."

—ROBIN S. SHARMA

We are influenced by peers and strangers hundreds of times each day. Due to social networks and our new way of consuming and digesting news the choice is diluted, and clarity has been slightly compromised.

Let's be honest, the days of food advertising on TV are over.

I remember being ten years old, tiny, loud and Italian (only one of these things has changed) and watching endless adverts for food on TV. Depending on the time of the day, the advert would target different age groups or specific foods. Almost twenty years ago, television was still the best way to see what was new, and celebrity endorsements were the most reliable way to catch people's attention. I could pretty much quote word by word a very specific Canned Tuna advert, simply by its' jingle. I do not remember the name of the brand, but the song, oh boy, it was catchy.

Back then though, the system was simple: once the product was ready to be produced marketers would buy a lot of TV ads, as well as billboards and magazine features. The ads would lead to retail distribution and sales.

Nowadays, things are slightly different. Catching attention is vital because we are impatient, and tend to lose interest quickly.

Statistics in the year 2000 showed that our average attention span for engaging with an advert only lasted a mere twelve seconds. This dropped to just eight seconds in 2013 (just one second below that of a goldfish, lucky us).[4]

Living in the information age, there are so many things vying for our attention; such as Instagram notifications, messages and group chats and an endless, pouring stream of GIFs.

This outpouring of information means that we have to make frequent, rapid decisions on whether we want to engage with something or not. This is where the old principle of peer review came back into fashion. It's not necessarily something that disappeared either.

Peer review is a great marketing tool, and you can easily find examples on a lot of websites: recipe websites (as well as Pinterest nowadays) encourage people to post photos of their finished meals. Fitness programs and Instagram accounts encourage 'before - and - after' photos so people can show others how much better they look.

The traditional economic theory argues that we make choices based on quality and price.[5] In this system of thought, it's claimed that if external influences have any effect, it's the one of having us follow others' lead in our choices. In this case, their reviews and opinions.

But there's another force at play, which comes with the saturation of any given market. I like to call it the snob effect. This refers to the fundamental principle that the more the general population likes something, the less interested the majority becomes.

It may sound like an oxymoron in itself, however, there is a bigger truth emerging here and that is that selected influence is key.

People value where they place their influence. Let me explain: the general public is looking for reviews, as well as recommendations from people they respect and aspire to be like.

This is where influence became, at first, an ingenious way for brands to send complementary products to bloggers and wannabe content creators.

Slowly things have changed in a way where the influencers have recognised the value of their work. The industry is growing at an unprecedented rate, meaning that influence is now almost seen a service that can be rendered.

As we started seeing it more and more as a service, we lost track of where influence comes from, and how it can really help.

Made to be influenced?

"Our minds influence the key activity of the brain, which then influences everything; perception, cognition, thoughts and feelings, personal relationships; they're all a projection of you."

—DEEPAK CHOPRA

This is going to blow your mind.

Someone has influenced almost every decision you have ever made. Whether it be the bartender looking to upsell their products, your friend boasting about their new hair drier or the stranger online who keeps banging on about this new almond milk that they are using in their porridge. Either way, they all played a part in your decision to buy, eat, shop, drink etc....

Social influence is not breaking news - look at my bibliography for proof. In the past, it has been mainly been used to influence whom we vote for, which energy provider we choose to what bank we sign up to. However, since traditional advertising has been in constant decline, and peer influence has slowly moved to the online world, the way we are influenced has changed.

Let's take Pip & Nut, for example; a nut butter company making waves in the world right now.

I met the founder Pip and right-hand-man Tom when they were just starting out; just a three-person team in East London. I have never really lost track of their activities, and have been witnessing their growth almost subconsciously.

First, they ended up being at every event I'd go to (and trust me, I go to loads of events). Their toast bar with the fiery red toaster shining in the distance. I would see their tubs lying in flat-lays alongside porridges, pancakes and smoothies.

Then, last December, I received a package from Pip & Nut with all of the essentials for a cosy winter night in: socks, mug and nut butter (of course).

Fast forward to a few weeks back, wandering in the supermarket in the spread section, I am looking for some nut butter - yes, I somewhat did run out. The choice is much bigger than a few years back, but among all the labels one catches my attention.

Which one?

You're damn right I chose Pip & Nut.

Why? Because I've seen my friends posting about it and I've seen strangers that I stalk online talking about it. Not to mention, the mug they sent me (with the socks for a winter night in) reminded me of it.

Because we are looking at relatable content, and relatable people, we are exposed to their decisions 24/7. So, does this mean that being online has turned us into highly-impressionable beings?

Not necessarily. The truth is that we have been looking for things to influence us all along.

Beyond the screen, social media and online world: influence is in our DNA.

We're influenced by others in everything we do, even if we're not aware of it; from imitating somebody word-for-word or doing the exact opposite of someone else just to be different.

Others are always guiding our actions.

Underneath it all, it's all about the simple, subtle ways that others affect our behaviour.

The good news is, the more we understand the topic of influence, the better we can handle it and just accept it as part of who we are.

We are made to be influenced, so much so that influence is constellating the world around us.

"Just like atoms bouncing off each other, our social interactions are constantly shaping who we are and what we do." *(Jonah Berger, Invisible Influence).*[6]

In fact, this pull toward the familiar goes so far beyond what we have currently discussed. For example, in the wake of big hurricanes, parents often give their children names that begin with the same letter as the storm. In the aftermath of Hurricane Katrina, the child's name Kathy skyrocketed it popularity in New Orleans.

Why does this happen?

These parents prefer such names merely because they've been exposed to the sound of the letter so much.[7]

The same concept shapes the way we influence others in multiple ways; it's the rule of the seven interactions - basically one of the rules we live by as a company.

When clients and members of the community ask me what it really takes for someone to take action, I directly answer;

"The Magnificent Seven".

What can I say? I do appreciate a good name.

Now, I do wish I could remember where I first read about this, but unfortunately, I do not have a source for this one. Oh, besides from the fact that it works again and again and again.

You could argue, my Dear Reader, that this is much more than influence.

In this case, we may be talking about *persuasion.*

Are you ready to be persuaded?

Persuasion, unfortunately, does get a bad rep, but it is objectively the next logical step to be taken into account after influence takes place.[8]

Dr William Miller developed a very clear example of persuasion with *Cognitive Interviewing.*

Cognitive interviewing argues that you can use open questions to guide the interviewee to think about their behaviour, which is something you could almost see as persuasion in itself.

Persuasion, when put to good use, can be incredibly impactful on individuals. However, persuading groups is entirely different, and this is where influence becomes an art (and persuasion does not apply as much). Persuasion is still pretty much about what you want to achieve, rather than a genuine way to help others take actions towards their own desires.

Business owners can easily persuade an individual to buy a new product with a very enticing and luring email. Sales Reps can eventually grind down that one particular client to buy their products after endless follow-up calls (I am sure most have been 'victims' of this).

But influencing groups?

That's a whole different kettle of fish; which is, by the way, a remarkable expression.

Influencing groups is, honestly and humbly, an Art.

It has been shown that members of groups may develop unique patterns of thinking and interacting concerning leadership that cannot be fully explained by their personal attributes.[9] As Sandelands pointed out in a study regarding group culture, "groups include individuals, to be sure, but individuals do not constitute them. Instead, we see that the group is a life, a being unto itself with a dynamic of its own", (*Sandelands, 1998*).[10]

This research showed that a group consisted of a particular number of people connected to each other in some way, or to a leader and an idea.

If we look at things from this perceptive, we realise that group culture and belonging have been part of the human experience since the dawn of time.

Since we can remember, human beings have been part of groups, communities and tribes, with a shared interest and a way to communicate.

If we read between the lines, we'll see something exciting here.

Did you spot it?

Reread the previous paragraph.

Yes, go on.

Now you got it! Communities do not need to know who their leaders are to grow and sustain themselves. Without a leader, a community will find its leader. However, without an idea, the community does not fundamentally exist. Leaders embody the idea and keep it alive, and because of social media and the online world, communicating has been more accessible than ever, and leaders can establish themselves much more easily.

Relief, right?

You may be thinking now, "all right, Fab, so you're saying that all I have to do is strategize over how to make a leader out of myself, using the power of persuasion?"

Well, before you start opening psychology books and wearing beaker glasses (creating a rather peculiar cross between a mad scientist and Freud) let me tell you this;

No influencer has been sitting down reading bibliographies on sociology, psychology and business.

This may be the reason why some marketers are incredibly frustrated at how well influencers have been performing despite their supposed lack of marketing-related skills.

People will start creating emotional connections with them naturally, so much so that they will be picking up cues by merely looking at their *online presence* and making assumptions.

Once, a fellow influencer got asked how their cat was feeling, after sharing a few days previously that they had to take their pet to the vet. This stranger felt much invested in the wellbeing of the kitten (which was healthy, happy and proceeded to live a long life, in case you were wondering). However, more to the point, followers genuinely invest in you and your life.

The influencers, most of the time, have no idea why people follow them and like every human in this tiny round sphere, Influencers also get confused, frustrated and demotivated.

What I can tell you though, is that everything does happen for a reason and before we get to the main content of this book and begin talking about the habits that create great influencers then let me introduce you to the protagonists of this book: the influencers themselves.

Made to influence?

"99.9 percent of all decisions are shaped by others."

—JONAH BERGER, INVISIBLE INFLUENCE[11]

Who is the person that influenced you the most?

If you had to answer, hands down, without thinking who would you pick?

No, do not cheat.

Answer right now, out loud.

Go on, nobody will mind.

I am asking you this because, nowadays, we believe influence is something that has been shaped by our hyper-social lives. I do have loads of friends who inspire me and influence me daily. However, my answer will be, always and forever: my Grandad.

Fun fact about me as a baby: I did not trust men.

At all.

My mum used to joke about the fact I'd cry when a man was holding me for more than a few seconds. I did not trust men and did not like being around them, which is quite funny when I think that for most of my life I have always had more male friends than female friends.

However, little Fab, was very suspicious of everyone, aside from my biggest influencer, my Grandad.

Oh, I loved spending time around him.

The things that I learned, the things that I loved were all pretty much linked to him in some way.

I can safely say he profoundly influenced both my brother and myself.

I still remember fondly the afternoons spent with my Grandad hopelessly trying to teach me how to play tennis (needless to say, I was not bound to be the new Serena Williams).

However, he always encouraged me to be incredibly creative.

I remember he once found his old easel and paints so he got me a new set of brushes and a subscription to a painting magazine and I began to paint. Even all of these years later, I will still buy notebooks and draw for hours.

We would play the piano together and dance to Frank Sinatra for hours on end.

"Because music is just great", he would say.

Pure and simple.

My Grandad may never have drank a green juice, or ran a business, or used a computer. He did not *teach* me what I needed to know to be who I am now.

However, he *influenced* me more than I could have been.

And that, Dear Reader, is influence.

So, who are the influencers?

If my Grandad was an influencer, who are these God-like figures, travelling the world, swimming with the dolphins, living these wonderful lives we see on your Instagram account?

Influencers, a bit like celebrities, are no different from you. Actually, you are most likely an influencer.

Just please, stop picking your nose, it's not nice.

In recent marketing terms, to be an influencer all you need to get started is an online presence. I am talking about your Facebook profile (the one you may have not updated since 2005 and still has embarrassing photos of your fresher's week).

The next step to be an influencer is to share endorsements, opinions and overall advice.

And *Voila*.

You are, indeed, an influencer.

As simple as that.

However, I do believe the term influencer has been misused recently as it has now been used as a synonym for *Social Influencer, Content Creator, Entrepreneur*, or simply a *Blogger*.

The topic of influencers is not a new idea.

In fact, the idea of influencers as a tool has been adopted by brands to spread awareness around their products for years.

Just think about a good old fashioned infomercial with a celebrity endorsement.

In *The Tipping Point*, Malcolm Gladwell argues that vitality is driven, "by the efforts of a handful of exceptional people",[12] whom he calls *Mavens, Connectors* and *Salesmen.*

The people are your influencers.

Different people have the ability to influence the people around them, online and offline, in different ways.

Here are a few examples;

Lynda is a personal trainer, and she uses her social accounts to share workout videos. These inspire her clients as well as new potential clients into leading a more active lifestyle.

Is she an influencer?

Yes.

What about Tom. He plays rugby with his team every Saturday and shares online his newest finds from the farmers market every weekend?

Is he an influencer?

Ding-ding-ding!

Another Yes!

Remember Alan, your colleague from IT? The one who so passionately spreads the good word about your company (and always brings cake at birthdays because he secretly has a Google calendar reminder set up?)

Ladies and gentlemen, we do have a winner.

Another Influencer. Can you believe it?

I could go on, and on, yet the point remains the same;

Influence is not measured by numbers, metrics or data.

That is merely a way to turn influence into a product that are easier to sell. Influence is measured by the impact.

To paraphrase Peter Parker's Uncle, *with great influence comes great responsibility.*

Who has the most significant influence then?

If it's not really a matter of numbers.

The answer: *social influencers*

Social Influencers.

Who are *social influencers*?

At risk of going down the definition rabbit hole, *Social Influencers* are now a synonym for Social Media Influencers.

In the good old days, when psychology manuals had all the answers, social influence was associated with peer pressure, persuasion and the capacity to influence someone's emotions, opinions and behaviours.

Right now, social media and the online world are training our influence muscle, so it's quite fair to say that *Social Influencers* have earned their spot in the industry.

A lot of people are still relatively critical and sceptical about *Social Influencers*, which of course, can be very demoralising.

Nevertheless, just less than ten years ago you would never call yourself a *Life Coach* or a *Blogger* and expect people to understand: these people were the early adopters of new and upcoming trends.

The sad things about *Social Influencers* is that some of us have traded our mission for the metrics which will be addressed in Habit One. This has, unfortunately, disillusioned with the whole system.

Successful *Social Influencers* have found a way to escape the trap of tracing Numbers and Following and adopt the *Six Habits* to transcend the metrics.

Think about it as a very abstract *Holy Grail*, if you may.

Great *Social Influencers* value the responsibility of their opinion and the ripple effect that it creates. Some websites will help you calculate with an algorithm (no joke) how *Social Influencers* can actually have the same magnitude as the *Peer Influencers.*

Peer Influencers.

Remember our friend Tom? Alan from IT, or the soccer mom Tanya? These folks have an incredible power of influence.

First of all, they are much blunter that most of the social influencers mentioned above.

When weighing up their metrics (numbers of impressions, or an overall number of people that actually read and interact with their opinion) versus their impact, their influence is exponentially higher.

They are incredibly honest (I recommend you having a look through your local Sainsbury's Google reviews if you do not believe me), especially as their reputation is not conducive to the *leading versus compromising* conundrum I spoke about in my introduction.

When your reputation is not at stake, there is a considerable load that you shed off your shoulders, which also may make Tanya's opinion more genuine and authentic.

Overall, we trust the opinions of other peers rather than the opinions of far-removed individuals we cannot relate with.

Is this reflective of a very sceptical and cynical society?

Even if some may say that it is actually much simpler than that.

Let me explain with this very relatable example.

Psychologist Richard Moreland of the University of Pittsburgh asked four women (all equally attractive) to attend multiple sessions of a college class with other students.

The women were instructed to participate in zero, five, ten and fifteen sessions of the class, respectively.

At the end of the semester, the students are given pictures of the women and asked to rate them based on their looks.

Despite not being aware of having met any of the women, the majority of the class picked the woman who'd attended fifteen sessions.[13]

What the study seems to suggest is that we do subconsciously have a closer bond with familiar people; especially when we are not made aware of it.

Brand Champions

The Cambridge Dictionary describes *Brand Champions* as, "a manager who is responsible for creating and developing a brand and encouraging support for it, both inside and outside a company".[14]

When I talk about *Brand Champions,* I usually put *Social* and *Peer Influencers* into the mix.

These people can be employees, customers and ambassadors who really believe in a brand and are advocating it effortlessly to the world.

Most *highly influential people* will become, one way or another, *Brand Champions* of companies they associate themselves with.

From a study conducted by Jonah Berger in his book *Contagious*; "the average American engages in more than sixteen word-of-mouth conversations where they say something positive or negative about an organisation, brand, or product".[15]

An excellent example of *Brand Champions* are company employees.

Brand Champions are the ones who spread the brand vision and brand values.

They are the ones that are most likely to live and breathe a brand and want it to succeed.

A Brand Champion goes beyond a specific sponsored or monetary retribution and becomes a true champion who will seamlessly use a particular product in various instances on their everyday life.

This is where a *Brand Champion* becomes a great asset for companies, and where can be great holders of positive influence.

What is positive influence, really?

Influence has plenty of definitions, just like the ones that I sprinkled in these past chapters.

However, I think it's essential to clarify what *positive-influence* means in the context of this book.

In one way or another *highly influential people* have a positive influence on others.

People can influence for many reasons, by tapping into a variety of emotions and feelings: curiosity, jealousy, envy (which ties in with comparison, a well-known process that is also a reason that makes influencers someone others aspire to be).

Influence has been and can be applied to any problem or idea.

Where positive influence is genuinely making a difference is by getting ideas spread, helping people be, feel and perform better as well as being happier overall.

It's not just about spreading an idea but spreading a positive one.

To use a much more technical term, I believe that positive influence is at the core of what is called *Ethical*

Leadership. Ethical Leadership usually points to a leader who is affecting the conduct of its employees (tribe or community) by providing a series of positive social norms. These social norms typically involve being honest, caring, trustworthy.[16]

This can take form in the shape of a CEO who allows employees to have Mental Health days or the blogger who, by example, takes time for self-care and rejuvenation.

When reading various studies (that were mainly carried out on a poll of business owners, managers and executives), the differentiating factor between social influence and positive influence are staggeringly obvious.

Leaders who are committed to *positive influence* tend to be emotionally linked to a selfless and grandiose mission that is usually related to a very personal story.

Think about Ella Mills for example, and her *Deliciously Ella* brand.

Her brand is routed in her very personal story of her struggle to fight an illness and it slowly evolved from a Blog to an App and then to Delis and eventually an ever-so-growing range of products available in supermarkets.

You could look at someone like Ella and see her as the perfect example of the progression from social influencer to a highly influential entrepreneur.

All she did was harness her positive influence through products, services and ideas that can carry the potential of helping others to carry a healthier life.

Positive influence starts with the reason *why* you do the work you do; regardless of where you are going to go and how you are going to evolve.

Influencers perform incredibly well because they naturally create a positive, self-motivated and pro-active version of themselves.

Thankfully for us all, some specific patterns are shown in the data and I call them the *Six Habits*.

Behind the Six Habits

"I like people who shake other people up and make them feel uncomfortable."

—JIM MORRISON

Why this book? Why now?

Like a lot of emphatic people in this industry I am all about supporting others. I have a very intricate personal mental health story (especially when I first faced my life-long history of depression over six years ago). All of this made me ask myself what I was really good at.

I realised that since a very young age I felt like I was not really good at anything that seemed to translate into my career.

That was mostly because of the cycle of low self-esteem, as well as my patterns and behaviours where I'd try not to stand out because I didn't want to be seen.

After hitting rock bottom one day at work, I decided to change the way I looked at my health. I realised how important it was for me to start getting my energy back.

I went through the tumultuous process of trying various lifestyles and diets (including juice cleanses, raw vegan diet, vegan, paleo, yoga, the Law of Attraction, moon rituals and meditation).

Thanks to the work I did on myself, I found a space in the world and began putting myself out there, and I came to notice I was incredibly good at bringing people together.

In that transition time where I converted from cups of coffee and Top 40 hits to the green juices and Tony

Robbins audio programs, I changed career and became a Marketing & Business Coach for Health Entrepreneurs.

As a long-time blogger (from the times of LiveJournal and MySpace), I decided to create a free group on Facebook where bloggers from all over the world could talk about Kombucha and health products.

Four years (and a lot of experiments later) that same community has reached over 100,000 people from all over the world.

We organise and facilitate events worldwide and we have an online membership and magazine.

I love how so many people will share their stories about their physical and mental health and inspire others to do the same.

Because of the nature of the business, I would ask a lot of questions.

I knew which questions I should ask and how to ask them.

This is how I began to realise that the people interacting with my group had an incredible influence on their audience, and could really make a positive change.

Running a community is less about you, and more about your tribe.[17]

Once again, with my ability to bring people together and my main focus being keeping people inspired and motivated, the community grew naturally as it was a genuine pleasant place to be.

Once again, it all comes back to asking my group questions and sincerely wanting to hear their answers.

We'll discover later on that asking the right questions is a big piece of the puzzle when it comes to successfully influencing people.

As I kept facilitating more and more ways for the people in my group to meet, share and learn, I soon realised I had become one of them. I wasn't just the leader of the group but an active member too.

Was it possible that I could find one (or more) habits that would present time after time for how somebody could be a successful Influencer?

As a nerd at heart (and a genuinely curious person) I knew that data was much more effective than speculation.

Just as high performers and successful entrepreneurs follow certain rituals and develop habits, so do influencers and for the sake of my own mission I asked for help in the health and wellness industry. These interviews are shared throughout the book.

This is my way to give back to all the people who believed in my vision and supported it from day one.

This is also my way to inspire them all to keep on going.

This book comes from the need to re-shift priorities in the world of social influence and encourage you to use your influence for something bigger than yourself.

If you are reading this, there is a very high chance some names on the back of this book really caught your attention.

"If he/she made it, how can I become the next [insert name]?"

I hope that you'll be able to realise that you do not need to become anyone else to achieve greatness.

However, you'll need to start with the drive to make a substantial difference in other people's lives. If you do not feel that borderline obsessive drive to be a trailblazer and a rule changer then this book may not be for you right now.

However, if you do you feel the need to make other people happier and want to the catalyst for something great then you're holding the right book in your hands. We live in a world where we have the influence to make things happen, conduct services that we believe in (especially in a marketplace that is begging us to make an impact) and yet, we still get stuck.

Here's where the six habits come into place.

How to read this book
(a note on semantics)

A few notes on definition and words:

- As I explained previously, there are quite a few different kinds of so-called influential people. In this book, when talking about *influencers,* I am specifically talking about *social influencers*.

- In the book I will layout out the different habits of successful Influencers in different sections. These Habits will be number One to Six.

- Throughout the book, you'll be able to find specific case studies from fellow influencers. They will be named and credited accordingly throughout.

The research for this book focused on two very different areas; *highly influential people* and *social influencers*. *Highly influential people* were a selected number of Influencers that I considered to be leaders in their field.

Most of them have books, successful collaborations and partnerships as well as businesses of their own. Some of these Influencers offered to answer some specific questions about their journey.

Very similar questions were asked to another group (the *social influencers*). These people are part of my wonderful community, and I was incredibly stoked by their willingness to take part in this.

Both questionnaires included various questions related to each and every one of *the habits*.

The aim of this research was to nail down the common patterns that shaped the influence of *highly influential people* (as well as outline the pain points of people still struggling to get there). These patterns shape our desires and beliefs for ourselves and for the world.

PART TWO:
THE SIX HABITS

At the core of the habits, some concepts and ideas are not necessarily new. Whenever I do a talk or host a panel, I clearly point out that we rarely re-invent the wheel; whether it's a product (see Seth Godin's *Purple Cow* for more) or an idea, being remarkable is not a by-product of genuine novelty.

These habits will not require you retreat to Tibet or go soul-searching. They all come with specific questions and implementations to allow you to follow through and take-action. These are also known as *keystone habits*.

These habits provide small wins, meaning early successes that are relatively easy to attain. Achieving the keystone habits helps you believe that change is possible.

Just like the famous Hero's Journey, it comes down to having a mission, a diverse set of skills and an expertise in a certain topic.

Habit One is all about your Goal, your Mission and your Story.

We'll explore why having a compelling reason behind your mission can inspire influence and leadership. We will look at how fear is not as scary as you might think and look at what Campbell's Hero Journey Theory can teach us about human behaviour. Finally, we will look at how a Doctor has found meaning through her personal story.

Habit Two shows you how to think like an entrepreneur and why you should start thinking about your future (and how to plan your next steps) like a BOSS! We will explore the idea behind being your own product, and why you should not rely on another platform to expand your portfolio. Furthermore, we'll discuss the subtle art of *driving for daylight*, as well as the rules of collaboration and partnership.

Habit Three explores the connection between credibility, trust and owning your content by providing the best information. We'll discuss the idea of remarkable marketing and the responsibility that comes with it. We will then look at the changes that have taken place in how the public view online experts.

Habit Four is one of my personal favourites, and it revolves around your Tribe. We will look at why being a leader is essential for your own influence, and how you can nurture your tribe by giving back. We'll also discuss why people need tribes, and how communities shape us up as a species.

Habit Five encourages you to never stop growing and learning, in order to maintain credibility and trust from your community. People tend to believe growing influence is a checklist you go through once and forget. In reality, influence is very closely linked to our ability to grow and develop (as well as admit our mistakes).

Habit Six is about your personal growth and preservation. Self-care and self-love have had a rebrand in recent times, and it is now a widely and openly discussed topic. This habit looks at how resting, reassessing our goals and moving forward will allow us to sometimes step away from the spotlight of influence and *just be*.

So, what's next?

Let's be honest, if your life is worth living then it's worth recording so let's start by making the decision to keep a journal and write by hand.

Why?

Because writing by hand boosts your memory.

When we write by hand, we have to coordinate both excellent verbal and movement systems. For example, at school or in the workplace we don't write verbatim, which means we have to create our own summaries and concepts. It only takes looking back over previous notes you've made to see how you have invented your own code to boost your memory.[18]

Personally, I've kept journals my whole life. I even used to have a *shared-secret-diary* with my best friend where we would write about our days and then swap for the other one to read.

This might be extreme, however, creatives, writers and thinkers all seem to have a writing routine of sorts. I know you'll find real value in putting your thoughts, ideas, and emotions on paper; there's a certain level of clarity that comes from journal writing that's difficult to reach any other way.

So get a fresh new notepad (go on, treat yourself) and make sure you jot down ideas, exercises and tips to really harness *The Habits.*

Get ready to join me on a riveting adventure; the kind of journey that you'd want to take your Polaroid on. The kind of journey that will make you cry, laugh and pretty much leave you exhausted by begging for more adventure.

I'll be sharing a lot about myself and my own journey, as well as sharing stories about my online community and the incredible people around me who have made this book possible.

There will be a lot of footnotes and books, research and studies mentioned along the way.

I am a geek after all.

Oh, and quotes.

There will be loads of quotes.

I always found quotes one of the most fascinating parts of a book. Therefore, to get things started allow me to quote Jimmy Wales (founder of *Wikipedia*):

"imagine a world in which every single person on the planet is given free access to the sum of all human knowledge. That's what we're doing."

Habits, not traits

"Excellence is an art won by training and habituation. We do not act rightly because we have virtue or excellence, but we rather have those because we have acted rightly. We are what we repeatedly do. Excellence, then, is not an act but a habit."

—ARISTOTLE

Once upon a time, I dreamed of being a music journalist. I had loved music my entire life; all thanks to my dancing session with my Grandad, and the sing-along session I had with my Mum in the car. Without realising it, my love and passion for music had become part of my daily routine. I was the weird ten-year-old who started making VHS mixtapes and spent hours recording MTV just to watch it again and again. Shortly afterwards I started reading music magazines and years later books about music.

They are small practices, which may be overlooked at first but they led me to my big breakthrough (my butterfly effect moment, if you may); the small steps that led me to where I am today.

I started writing articles and sent them to magazines. The first ever series that I had published online was a three-piece essay about the correlation between the Doors and literature.

I still remember those three articles, and how proud I felt of myself and without those articles I would not be where I am today.

Those small rituals made me who I am today, in a way that I could not predict. I was not born with any musical talent, I was just doing things again, and again for my enjoyment. These were not traits, but practices.

I am a Virgo, which some people believe to be a clear indicator of patterns of my behaviour, and some other people do not really buy into. Nevertheless, very Virgo-like traits I possess include tidiness, a very peculiar fascination with storage, binders and organisers among others.

Those are traits - and their limiting nature is linked to the idea that it entails a quality or characteristic belonging to one person.

Habits go one step further, thanks to their triggers as cognitive psychologists define them as "automatic behaviours triggered by situational cues"[19] - which translates as things we do with little or no conscious thought.

Habits are practices

Let's say you are sitting at the dinner table with your family one night, and all of a sudden, your sister from the other side of the table sneezes. What is the first instinct of everybody else around the table?

"Bless you."

What can be seen as politeness is, objectively, a habit: an action repeated so frequently that it's now processed unconsciously in your brain.

Research shows that one way our brain saves energy is by creating habits - some studies indicated that as many as 40% of the actions you perform each day are based on habits and patterns and not on conscious decisions.[20] This is also the reason why a research study shows that we follow our habits when willpower is low - this can be when we naturally have 'low willpower' or something has happened in the day to reduce it.[21]

Habits tend to be regular, or somewhat settled. They may develop from heritage and mimicking, or discipline. Nevertheless, there is some sort of commitment - whether intentional or not - that shapes a habit.

The truth is, products do shape our habits as well through their essence as, when used habitually, they can alter our everyday behaviour.[22] Behaviour and habit are fascinating concepts that genuinely dictate who we are and what we do.

If habits are a way of behaving, than traits can be considered habits in themselves. However, habits tend to be born out of necessity, or a desire. They also are linked to our beliefs and patterns, which can be changed and influenced.

Just think about the hours spent reading motivational and self-help books (smashing that fourth wall again) and how reading a book like this may change some of your current habits. By being able to recognise patterns and beliefs, habits can be cultivated and can help - in this particular case - to harness and grow social influence.

You may be wondering - would people ever capitalise on habits?

Hell to yeah!

(Excuse my enthusiasm back there)

Habits are something that is extensively studied by marketers and retailers to adapt their operations to maximise sales - and you'll be surprised by what they can pick up: most people instinctively turn right when entering a store; therefore, retailers put their most profitable products on the right side of the entrance.[23]

If marketers are using our habits for their own benefit, how can we do the same?

How to cultivate habits

You may already know me in person. If so, oh lucky you. But if you do not, you may come across something about me - probably from the first second you meet me. I am incredibly excitable (read, impatient). If anything, it can be incredibly flattering to dog, sloth and cute baby owners.

My point is, when we learn things that excite us, we tend to become really impatient. As you are flicking through the book, you may be tempted to implement everything as you go along. Do not worry, it's incredibly common, I have been there myself - and it's something I am learning to be more mindful of.

This book is chock-full of habits, and habits need to be cultivated. Just picture the habit as a seed. A tiny seed dropped in the soil. You first get excited and decide to water it once. For the first week, actually, you are being incredibly attentive. Then, as days go by, you see new seeds and start planting them - forgetting about the old seed.

Habits are much easier to maintain than to cultivate, so once something becomes a habit, you can shift your discipline into forming a new one and then build them up sequentially. This doesn't just tackle your ability to cultivate habits, but it also trains selective discipline. Selective discipline is what allows you to form enduring good habits, while immediate, explosive discipline will work best for bursts of energy. The habit itself is not enough, selective discipline will help you endure and reap the benefits.

If you want to cultivate a habit, make time for it.

Habits are relatively easy to dissect: you have a trigger, or cue, to which a particular routine act follows, and lastly the reward and once your brain registers the successful completion of the activity it will reinforce the link between the cue and routine.

Studies show that our brain is anticipating the reward even before we get it, and by denying the actual compensation we may get frustrated and mopey. This is the neurological basis of craving.[24]

Do you ever catch yourself checking your email for the hundredth time only to discover that, still, nothing exciting has arrived in your inbox?

This process is known as "partial reinforcement extinction effect" (a bloody long name I know) - what this really means is that you keep repeating the same action, even without reward, simply because you're used to doing it unrewarded.

To cultivate habits, you must be able to understand how to implement it and feed that craving sensation - it comes down to practice as well as clear ways to measure your improvements.

Cultivating a good habit is ultimately a way to make it almost second nature - something you want to harness not just for the toolkit I'll be sharing with you in the course of this book, but overall in your daily life.

Habit One: Have a Mission that Feels Uncomfortable

Be a storyteller

I remember that day as if it were yesterday.

I was so excited since I had my first book right in my hands. I've been writing it for so long, I remember thinking about the structure, the short stories, and the actual flow of the whole book.

It was a collection of horror stories and poems I wrote throughout the years and transcribed from my paper notepad into my first laptop. Looking back, it was the first time I had shown some entrepreneurial skills. I took something I 'd fallen in love with and worked hard for it.

Just like all the best stories, mine started at a library - ever seen The Breakfast Club?

This may come as a surprise, but I have always been a bookworm. I mean, a really fast reader as well. So much so that when I went to the library, while on vacation, and discovered in sheer horror, it was going to be closed for *two consecutive days*, I stacked up 11 Goosebumps books, marched to the checkout, and looked at the librarian.

"This is the first time someone reaches the allowance of daily books to book out" she said.

A greedy smile tinted my face. Nevertheless, my greediness came back to bite me right in the bum when a few days later I came back with all of my books (there was not much to do aged 10 before the Internet was a thing) and nothing more to read in the kids' section.

So I braved it up, and there I was, aged 10, heading to the grown-up section of the library. Trust me, I was a bit intimidated. Would I find something that would really excite me? How could anything feed my lust for horror and weird stories?

So, as I was walking about, right at my eye level, I spotted a book that actually caught my attention. There it was, with its bright, surreal cover: it was Stephen King's *Desperation*; the bright and quirky cover really spoke to me.

I picked it up, and just like in the best love story, I knew it was the one.

For the rest of the summer, I read dozens of Stephen King's novels and short stories. The more I read, the more I knew that was what I wanted to do. If he could do it, why would I not be able to?

So the first story of my first book was written on a yellow pad with a pencil, smudging most words as I went along - on reflection probably not one of my smartest moves.

There and then I knew I wanted to be a writer.

My mum, a couple of years later, surprised me with my first collection of short stories, which I still own to this date. That was my first book.

This is the story of how I decided I was going to be a writer.

How stories shape our perception

Stories really change the world; I've seen it myself. The reason why influencers can influence is because they are relatable. Stories make you relatable because you can speak very directly to each and every one of the people you are touching - just like a Meta writer would break the fourth wall again and again.

Anyone can tell and learn from a story, as storytelling has been the primary method for imparting knowledge since we can remember. In fact, our receptivity towards stories does come from somewhere.

Stories have been the way for our ancestors to gather and share essential information. You can imagine a group sitting around a stone cave, listening intently to a man talking about his fight with a big bear right next to the river. They all take it in, each and every one of them, learning and processing. They are captivated, but they are also learning something. Stories like this have information and some educational value: for example, if you are going next to the river, you better bring a sharp stick.

This is speculated to be the reason why, when a good story captivates us, the neurotransmitter dopamine is released in the brain, which causes our concentration and interest to heighten.[25] People don't just share information: they tell stories, as stories are vessels that carry morals and lessons.

Stories are the best way for us to learn something new.

Before the printing press made mass distribution possible, most information was shared orally - which is part of the reason why the stories grandparents tell us are always the most memorable.

I still remember the story my Grandad told me about when he was just a child, in the time of the fascist regime. Every year they had a parade running through the main street in his town, were soldiers and important people of the administrations would be praised.

Once, he sneakily got to the front of the line, holding the fresh bread he bought from the shop. He started throwing loaves to the fascist soldiers, trying to hide himself in among the crowd.

As they spotted him, they started running after him, but he eventually managed to flee. It was one of the favourite stories of his, which I will always remember.

A truthful and very well told story is what really can make you stand out from the crowd.

When we listen to a story, our brains process the information just like they process real life[26] – pretty cool that brain of ours, huh? By telling your own story, you are already creating a character that people can relate to: yourself. There is an arch, development if you may, that is part of what it is to be a human being.

There is a lot of talk about authenticity nowadays, but I think authenticity comes naturally when you're staying true to yourself and what your story is really about.

So how can you make your story stand out, and why should you?

The reason why it is – and it comes down to our information overload – is because we are inundated by information wherever we go. Despite being incredibly helpful to instil credibility, it's quite difficult to remember an isolated statistic or fact. However, according to psychologist Jerome Bruner, if these pieces of information are put into a story, we're 20 times more likely to remember them.[27]

Our brain is always trying to assess information that is given to it, especially because in order to be focused on one matter we need to keep our dopamine levels high. Every second, our brains are juggling with around 11 million pieces of information coming from our senses, yet we can only process between five and seven (not talking millions here) of them.[28]

If facts are not enough to hook us, how can we tell compelling stories?

Relatable and emotional connection are a very crucial aspect of compelling stories. Just like fiction writers need to put you in their protagonists' shoes, harnessing the power of strong emotions is critical - and is also what creates vitality in the online world. Coming back to the idea of real life and fictional connecting, when we know what the protagonist is doing, like chasing a bear with a stick, for example, the same areas of the brain are activated as if it were we who were doing the action.

A lot of bloggers within our community worry about choosing the right topics, and finding out *what* the reader wants to hear, forgetting about *how* they want the reader to feel: indignation? Excited? Terrified?

Those feelings create a strong emotional connection that gives stories longevity.

A simple, yet effective example of this is Metro's *Dumb Ways to Die* song-come-advert, so subtle that when the message hits you, you've been lured into a false sense of comedic security. Teaming up with infamous gaming brand *Dumb Ways to Die*, the 2012 campaign features a few examples of common accidents happening in and around trains, playing at first on the audiences' feeling of disgust and despair, while successfully highlight the importance of rail safety. The song has received over 170m YouTube views to-date.[29]

You might be asking yourself, quite rightfully, how can I do this, especially when I'm not writing a whole novel?

To craft a great story, you need context, action and the result (CAR). And what's true for academics is as true for influencers. A lot of people can get hung up on the context. When you're establishing context, it's important that you try your best to ensure that your audience can relate to your story as much as possible.

This means that, when telling a story, make sure that you have a clear point you are trying to put across. All you have to do is create a good mixture of success and failure, as well as aiming to give back to your audience by providing them with something tangible that they can act on themselves because of the conclusion to your story.

What I am trying to say is that you do not have to make up anything. Just practise your story-telling skills.

The word-count of your stories will not stop you from creating an incredibly engaging piece of content. Even a caption can have an incredibly strong story, and that is mainly due to the combination of story and visual. Indeed creating a visual connection can help to strengthen a story, and that is very much related to the immediate impact images have.

Take advertising for example; a lot of those are simply very short stories that amaze the viewers, some of them in ways you'd not expect.

Imagine a boy in a tennis court, against an adult. They are about to play a match, and your expectations are all set. The boy looks like he is scoring all the points. It's unusual and surprising, and therefore piques the viewer's interest. As the viewers are confused, they keep watching to the end because they want to know why the little boy is so good. In the end, it is revealed that he is the son of tennis players Steffi Graf and Andre Agassi.

This old advert is one of my favourites: it uses a twist to keep you hooked.

A very strong use of your storytelling skills, stories, especially the ones told through a very specific mix of formats, will allow you to tap into different types of learners simultaneously - in fact, 40% of us are visual learners, 40% are auditory learners and the remaining 20% are kinaesthetic learners.

However, a well-constructed story will attract all three: imagery influences visual learners, vocabulary appeals to auditory learners and the emotions conveyed connect with kinaesthetic learners. Especially when carefully placed, they can trigger some associations our brains will be wanting to replicate - and funnily enough, most of us do not even know why.

This is the reason why social media and other platforms, harnessing some specific analytics, can validate our speculations on whether a specific piece of content has been successfully received by our audience.

99% of the time, a key aspect of storytelling will be part of the content.

Motivating people to share stories with one another is the best way to build up strong relationships within a tribe. All *highly influential people* are incredibly powerful storytellers, in one way or another.

How to become a better storyteller

I have a confession to make: I love going to the App Store and literally start wondering around, looking for new apps to try. I am a geek after all. One of the latest apps to get my full attention was featured in the App Store a while back, and it's called Quartz.

Quartz acts like an edgy news reader in your pocket, in the form of text messages sent to your phone - yes that includes GIFS and emoji's. Digestible nuggets to keep you in the loop - definitely targeting millennials, too busy to spend hours on BBC News apparently.

If we just ignore the positive and negative implications in the realm of journalism, Quartz pretty much summarises how people, in general, are consuming, digesting and repurposing content these days - says, writing endless posts on her blog. In a world of bullet lists and 3-step solutions, we are more and more surrounded by quick haikus or information (marketing, blogging, health).

From 140 characters to 24h pieces of content, there are only two possible avenues we can go down - I don't believe there is such a thing as right or wrong.

Avenue no. 1: Let Information be a Haiku

Let information be bite-sized. I mean, we can even buy Kit Kat minis - if that's not a sign, I don't know what that is. After years and years of blog posts telling us that 5000-word articles are the way to go, concise and pragmatic writers will rejoice by knowing that the audience in 2016 digs short, inspiring, and straight to the point insights. That said, your blog has a great deal of competition (especially when you think of Facebook and Instagram).

Nevertheless, you can become an expert in your field by simply becoming a medium of information (a bit like Quartz does) and commenting on the latest trends, rather than writing verbose how-to articles.

If you think I am being biased, you couldn't be further from the truth. I am probably the most verbose human being you'll meet at a dinner party - I warned you - so I definitely do not reside in this Haiku category. However, I find it interesting how quick opinion pieces, mixed with unicorn GIFS, are becoming more and more the norm.

Avenue no. 2: The BBC news of Blogging

This is more where I reside, I guess. To be honest, I did launch an online magazine - let me repeat that - an online magazine.

"Oh, that sounds like a fun side hobby" people would comment.

As it takes us around 20 hours per week to draft, proofread, schedule and review the Goddamn thing, so we'd better not call this a hobby.

Dragging myself back from the tangent, despite the hard work, I do believe in the power of editorial - of informed and researched articles that have something to say.

In the age of big online publications feeding you 12 takes on the Low-Carb diet each, and every month (I did check, for the love of research), information overload has its downfalls.

Don't get me wrong, I do not have anything against these publications - however, I am much more of a fan of longer, researched, in-depth articles that come from reliable sources. Well-thought editorial, engaging and interactive.

Personally speaking, I am not using one single technique to reach my audience, but I am instead combining different techniques in order to maximise the reach depending on what people need, and ultimately what I do enjoy.

One thing you cannot negotiate on is the ability to tell an engaging and convincing story. It is an art that requires training such as going to the gym would do ? It can also make you a powerful influencer, as it taps into the power of persuasion.

When it comes to practising your story, I recommend you take your story out for date: I love networking events for this sort of exercise.

Find an event that looks enticing enough, and go there on your own (come on, I know you can do it). After introducing yourself to other people in the room, practise telling people about your mission and how you are planning to make an impact. The more you practise your story asking others questions about themselves, and incorporating direct experience, the better you will become at influencing others.

On becoming comfortable with being Vulnerable: Michelle Elman from Scarred not Scared

Michelle Elman is an incredible human, speaker and writer very passionate about activism and body positivity. We discussed storytelling, public speaking and someone's voice as Michelle remarks that telling stories is part of everything she does: "my public speaking is solely storytelling".

Why do you think stories engage and resonate with people much more than other ways?

I think humans are innately captivated by stories since caveman periods when storytelling was a vital way to communicate. It has also been scientifically shown that storytelling activates more of our brain. In addition, I feel stories are more encompassing as each audience member is able to take away their own learnings without being prescribed a takeaway message.

Do you think that relatability has a place in this? How is the online world amplifying that in your opinion?

I think stories often help us feel less alone and with platforms like Instagram, we are able to find proof that we aren't left alone quite easily. Merely looking for the hashtag or googling the problem you have, will surface thousands of accounts and blogs with endless information and tools and I think that's really beautiful.

How do you think your voice has evolved online, and do you believe writing longer, more engaged captions was part of it?

My voice has definitely evolved over the last 4 years, simply because I have evolved and my captions reflect that. Especially in the last 2 years, I have found freedom in expressing my thoughts via writing. I personally find writing long captions therapeutic and more interesting as I am able to engage in more complex issues and discuss the nuance within each section.

What do you think makes a good writer?

I don't know if I would ever categorise myself as a good writer, but what made me eventually sit down and start writing my book was because I realised my grammar and spelling was not as important as my message. I had something to say, and if I didn't say it, those words and those thoughts would die with me and so that's why I started writing. Is my writing error-free nowadays? No. But if it conveys a message, then it served its purpose.

Is writing good compelling stories something that can come with practice?

I definitely think practice does help, but it's not so much to do with the story-telling but becoming more comfortable being vulnerable. Over the years, my confidence grew, and that's what really helped my storytelling - I felt braver to tell stories that could potentially be seen as controversial.

How good stories can go from paper to an audience via the medium of public speaking?

Through public speaking, I only use stories for the same reason I believe in storytelling on the page, that the audience is able to take away whatever message they need. You can tell a story in a room of 100 people, and each person will have a different take away depending on what they need in that moment or what applies to them, and I think that's why it's more impactful. No-one is ever moved or remembers a good PowerPoint presentation, people do remember a good story though.

Repetition is the mother of skills

"The repetition itself becomes the important thing;
it's a form of mesmerism"

—HARUKI MURAKAMI

Back to my old Tony Robbins cassette tapes; one of the sayings that will be stuck in my mind until my very last day is the old *repetition is the mother of skills*. Because, well, it is. Storytellers find that they have a lot to say, but not necessarily a lot of time to say it.

Despite being slightly annoying when your grandad keeps repeating the same thing again and again, repetition is essential to get my writing done, especially when taking the time to create content may feel daunting at times.

When it comes to routines, habits and ways of shaping life around your mission, different people throughout history have experimented with different approaches. I will be using artists and creatives as my main example, as I find that most of them can be incredibly relatable to people often engaging in the "side hustle" on a tight schedule.

Although no one consciously chooses difficult life circumstances, there are some influencers (in different industries and areas of trading) who choose to have little free time or to keep their day jobs in order to pay the bills.

When it comes to routines, I love snooping around writer's routines (I do believe they are the most regimented and overall fascinating).

Let's start with a little extract stolen from a Kurt Vonnegut a letter to his wife in 1965:[30]

> *"In an unmoored life like mine, sleep and hunger and work arrange themselves to suit themselves, without consulting me. I'm just as glad they haven't consulted me about the tiresome details. What they have worked out is this: I awake at 5:30, work until 8:00, eat breakfast at home, work until 10:00, walk a few blocks into town, do errands, go to the nearby municipal swimming pool, which I have all to myself, and swim for half an hour, return home at 11:45, read the mail, eat lunch at noon. In the afternoon I do schoolwork, either teach or prepare. When I get home from school at about 5:30, I numb my twanging intellect with several belts of Scotch and water ($5.00/fifth at the State Liquor store, the only liquor store in town. There are loads of bars, though.), cook supper, read and listen to jazz (lots of good music on the radio here), slip off to sleep at ten. I do push-ups and sit-ups all the time, and feel as though I am getting lean and sinewy, but maybe not. Last night, time and my body decided to take me to the movies. I saw The Umbrellas of Cherbourg, which I took very hard.*

To an unmoored, middle-aged man like myself, it was heart-breaking. That's all right. I like to have my heart broken."

Author Haruki Murakami, whose quote can be found at the beginning of this section, ran a small jazz club in Tokyo for several years before his career gained momentum. Once his writing career kicked off, he chose to move to a rural area and craft his own routine: waking at 4 a.m., working for five or six hours, running or swimming in the afternoon, then listening to music and reading before falling asleep at 9 p.m.

When talking repetition, I think rituals, routines and practises that do shape our habits. Goals and visions do have something in common: repetition, routines and questions.

Rituals and routines are something that can be supported with a few key tools - which I am definitely experimenting with since writing this book. The beauty of a routine is that it will affect people differently.

On the one hand, writer Toni Morrison, for example, likes to rise at around 5 a.m. to see the sunrise. For her, it's important to wake before the light and observe the transition into the day, tapping into her writing inspiration. On the other hand, Ann Beattie is what you'd call a night owl, working most productively from 12 a.m. to 3 a.m.

Some people can be such morning people that, well, they cannot get enough.

Novelist Nicholson Baker, for example, reaps the benefit of two mornings in one day by waking up for his first writing session at 4 a.m., then going back to sleep, and rising once again around 8:30 a.m. for his second-morning streak.[31]

Personally speaking, I always aim to go to bed quite early as I am a morning person.

Someone asked me in the past when I like to work out, and objectively, in an ideal world, I would always work out after work. This is mainly because mornings are my creative time, and THAT is my priority. I believe that forcing yourself to be a "morning person" or a "night owl" is just counterproductive in the long run. Make the most of your most productive for things you want to prioritise. It's unlikely I'll skip a class, but very possible I will not get to sit down and write if I do not have enough time in the morning, before hitting emails and general biz endeavours.

At the end of the day, there are a lot of techniques that can be used to keep us accountable when working on our stories. Even more essential than routines, questions are what really can support us to make a greater impact.

Be an investigator

"Curiosity is one of the permanent and certain characteristics of a vigorous intellect."

—SAMUEL JOHNSON

My grandparents used to have loads of books, and loads of encyclopaedias. My Grandad loved doing crosswords and used the books to find answers to some questions her would not know the answers for.

My favourite book of the whole lot was the animal encyclopaedia, the one about sea life, to be precise. I am not sure what that was: whether it was the fish, or the actual photos really enticed me; however, I would read it again and again and again.

I know, not the typical children's book, but I definitely wasn't the typical child. Once as I was reading the book mentioned above, my grandad came in, and I asked him a question about the clownfish to which he replied pointing at the caption.

"Why is he called the clownfish?" I asked.

He replied the best he could I suspect, by going with his instinct - he was not an expert in animals in any way, shape, or form.

"And why is *that the case*? "I asked again.

I'm saving you the whole story here, but I'm pretty sure it went along for about another five minutes. I did have this rather unappealing habit of asking *why* again and again and again, until in my tiny brain I thought I got to the bottom of it.

I was relieved years later to get to know that it wasn't just me. In fact, kids ask loads of questions to help them make sense of the world around them as they are just beginning to learn about it - it appears that children aged between two and five ask a total of some 40,000 questions.[32]

Researcher Brandy Frazier[33] found that pre-schoolers aren't asking questions merely as a way to seek attention, as they do care about the answers they receive. So much so, that a child is more likely to continue to ask "why?" when a parent's answer doesn't satisfy their thirst for knowledge.

Whenever you ask a question, you are focusing on the things you don't know - it's only once you know what you don't know, that you can think about how to fill the gaps in your knowledge. As adults, we forget that asking the right questions is the best way to get the right answers. By asking ourselves questions we actually get to think about problems at hand.

Indeed, asking ourselves questions is something that makes us unique as humans - have you ever seen a monkey asking themselves why they are monkeys? This is why great coaches always ask the right questions, or why some mindfulness – and minds at practices – are actually based on questions we ask ourselves in order to provide the answers.

Let's take the gratitude practice, all what it is, you answer the question of "what are you grateful for?" A very simple yet powerful tool. It is not a surprise that through my research I discovered that *highly influential people* ask themselves a lot of questions.

By deciding which questions we are going to ask ourselves we take power back into the decision-making of our lives. Incredibly successful people know how to harness powerful questions in order to solve difficult problems. *Highly influential people* tend to spend double the time questioning themselves and their choices than less influential people, which again proves my point that self-awareness a lot of the time is our response to very specific questions that we ask ourselves instead of living in autopilot.

So what questions should you ask yourself?

As we now know, questions are often linked to problems or gaps of knowledge that need to be filled.

In October 2007, graduates Brian Chesky and Joe Gebbia were trying to make a life for themselves in San Francisco.

They were struggling to pay their rent of $1150 and were faced with a simple choice: find a way to make more money, or go back home. Like in the best stories, this is when the penny dropped: the Industrial Designers Society conference was coming to San Francisco, and they knew there would be a shortage of hotel rooms, so they asked themselves: "*why do people have to stay in an overpriced hotel? Why couldn't we just offer a room in our place, for far a much better price*?"

They decided to rent out some space in their apartment where people could sleep on one of their three blow-up mattresses for $80 a night. They called this their *Airbed & Breakfast* and promoted it on design blogs with ads that focused on their apartment's features, like its "design library."

Airbed & Breakfast later became - I shall let you guess, Dear Reader - what we know as Airbnb this venture of renting three blow-up mattresses in a San Francisco apartment turned into thousands of people renting out their living spaces all over the United States, and subsequently, the whole world.

The right questions lead to the best outcomes - and most times, I find that the real change happens when you simply change your questions.

The fastest way to change what you're focusing on is to change the questions you're asking yourself.

Change from, "What happens if I fail at this?" or "Why do I always screw these things up?" to "What's the best way to get this done now?" or better yet, "What's the best way to get this done and enjoy the process?"

Taking the time to ask yourself meaningful questions in order to solve problems is key for both your core mission and anything you want to share with your audience. Not only, as mentioned before, asking questions becomes a tool to support clarity in your own path, but it also allows you to understand how you can help others most effectively.

This also proves that asking FOR questions is as important as asking the questions themselves.

Sometimes, the simplest questions can lead to a much unexpected solution: in 1944, a 3-year-old girl asked her father why she could not see the picture he had just taken of her. At the time, camera film was much different than what it is now, and the father knew it would have taken loads of time to develop the film. However, he decided to fulfil his daughter's wish - and this lead photographer Edwin Land work hard to find a solution to the unsatisfying answer, launching the Polaroid Land Camera in 1948.

How can influencers be tapping into questions? I find that most *highly influential people* take time to engage in Q&As, ask questions to their audiences or mailing lists, or join panels in order to really understand what their audience needs from them.

Once you know the questions, HOW you answer can be easily improved by learning how to tell a story that can facilitate your answer.

Why questions are within our nature

As humans, we tend to repeat our mistakes and fall into patterns - it's just the way we are wired since childhood. One of my most recurring patterns I would lovingly call *the juggler.* I am able to juggle thousands of things at once, ending up spreading myself too thin, feeling overwhelmed and burning out.

It used to happen more often than I would admit, and once it got really bad.

I was juggling business coaching, the first, new-born instance of the Health Bloggers Community and a Network Marketing business. At the time I was in a mastermind group with fellow biz ladies, and we would often have calls and check-ins.

I remember that day very clearly.

It was only two of us in that call, and I could already feel the tension growing inside of me. One of my dear friends (and someone I consider almost a mentor) Suzy was at the other end of the Skype call - we talked about respective struggles and hurdles, about stresses and fears, moving along to goals and aims.

She sensed my frustration: one question too many and I am in a puddle of tears (I am an incredibly emotional human, sloths can send me into a tailspin and have me sobbing from adorableness).

Once I regroup, she looks at me and, after the longest silence, she smiles at me and asks me.

> *"If you had a million pounds, right now, would you be doing what you are doing right now?"*

I remained speechless, for a good few seconds. I skimmed through everything I was doing, and it was clear a lot was meant to go. The network marketing business, the coaching. I wanted to grow the HBC to higher heights, I wanted to reach as many people as I possibly could with my message.

Everything else was not worth it. I was stuck in that limbo of doing what I am "meant to do" opposed to what I am "supposed to do".

When fear kicks in the right questions challenge you, help you to identify problems, find solutions and figure out how to turn solutions into reality.

Especially when fear strikes, questions can bring you back to a place of stability. Putting this very simply, we ask ourselves questions all the time, and this comes down to our focus: the way you feel and what you experience in your body comes from what you focus your attention upon during a given moment.

At any moment, you are "deleting" most of what is going on around you. That is, to feel bad, you have to delete (not focus on, not think about) everything that's great in your life. And vice versa.

For you to feel good, you have to delete the things you could feel bad about. This process of deleting is an important part of how the mind maintains the balance in one's emotional state. Undirected, however, it can wreak havoc in your day-to-day experience.

At this moment, how you're evaluating things determines what you focus on. Evaluations are nothing but questions you ask yourself. Your state, and ultimately, your life is the result of the questions you ask.

To manage your states via focus, you must control the questions you ask yourself. Eliminate limiting, "endless loop" questions. Continually ask yourself questions that empower you.

I am listing a few questions I always find extremely valuable, especially in moments of hardship:

1. What can I do today to get from A to B?

2. What have we not tried yet, to solve this problem?

3. What are all the benefits you'll gain by taking action?

4. How will this decision enhance your life?

What is fear anyway?

Fear is a series of unanswered questions.

If you find yourself still pretty much away from the highly-influential stage you're looking to reach, it's very likely there is one thing holding you back, and that is your own fear.

The essence of being successful at harnessing your leverage is being aware of your fear: over 80% of influencers interviewed agreed that they often take action despite fear. Because this fear is the fear of leading, and the fear of failing.

Interestingly enough the fear of failing is usually shaped by questions that stir from an endless list of "*What if?*"

It's a very powerful fear because you do not have to technically fail for the fear to set in. Failure in itself is not scary, let's be honest. It's the blame, the guilt, the criticism that may come with it. This is why a lot of us subconsciously decide to lay low - and touch enough people, without getting any criticism for it.

The truth is, you will fail. You will be criticised. Not everyone will like what you have to say, but you will spark a conversation. If you do not put anything out there, you'll never be able to start that fire. The answer to the question "*what should I do if I fail?*" is very simple.

Make it impossible for yourself to fail in the first place.

Failing to me is giving up, and hell I am not giving up, because I have a strong mission and a strong why to keep me grounded. Supporting people make an impact with their message is my mission, and if I manage to touch one person each and every single day, my work is done.

That is my succeeding - it's not ROI, it's not an income goal or a bunch of free classes. Those are targets that keep you accountable and allow you to enjoy life. It's so easy to fail when you make it really easy for yourself to fail. Both *highly influential people* and *social influencers* agree that they push themselves by acting outside of their comfort zone. However, 45% of *social influencers* stated that "*not knowing myself really well*" may affect their confidence.

By knowing yourself, your mission, your story very well you allow yourself to build the confidence to stand against criticism. To me, criticism is proof that we got people to think and react - remember: the things that get talked about are the ones that are worth talking about.

Why are you here?

Do you remember those days? The ones that get stuck in your memory, and you cannot shake them off? The ones that will change you forever?

I remember the day very well.

I just picked up my dad from the hospital. We are in the car, going back home. He starts feeling sick as we pull out of the hospital. I look at him, slowly getting out of the parking lot.

He looks at me, in his eyes, I can see he's hoping I won't say a word.

"We should get back. You are not well."

"I just want to go home."

"You are clearly not well."

My dad hated hospitals with a passion, yet he has been in and out for almost two years by that point. They agreed to release him provisionally, hoping his situation settled for the time being.

He keeps repeating "I just want to go home" again and again.

Tired and resigned, I make my way home.

An hour goes by, and I am lying on the floor in my own bedroom as my dad is in the bathroom, again, not able to stand up.

He is too heavy, and I cannot physically pick him up.

I told him we should have gone back, I told him he was not well enough.

I am alone, in my own house, lying on the floor, and I start crying.

I ask for help, and eventually, my aunt and uncle convince him to get back to the hospital.

That memory is just one symbolic moment of how I felt for a long time: that feeling of powerlessness, and intense deep sadness. I cannot do anything to help, there is nothing we can do, if not wait.

Fast-forward to October 2017: I am in a very unusual setting.

The sun is shining and I am sitting down on the porch in my room in Ibiza, looking at a question posed to me in a book, being almost confused by it.

The question in the book asks me to seek clarity. Find urgency. Redefine my why. I have not done that in quite a while. Then, like in all good stories, my why hits me like a well-placed front kick.

The truth is, I am petrified to ask myself why.

It's because of my dad, who battled with cancer for over seven years.

It's because of my grandma, who lived a life of medication and was not even been able to recognise me.

It's because one of my best friends, currently going through chemo once more.

My Why is not about me?

It's about my grandchildren, being able to play with nana in the back garden.

It's about my children, being about to think for themselves, be healthy and happy, and feel empowered to be exactly who they are meant to be.

It's about the impossible task of making the world better for others, in order for nobody to go through what I saw, and experienced, through the eyes of the people I loved.

It's about all of the incredible people with a strong influence, whose stories can change others without never meeting in person.

It's about a pain, a sadness I do not want anybody else to go through ever again - and being able to give others the tool to inspire a better, happier, healthier life to the world around us.

Whys can suck big balls, let me tell you that. However, whys are all around us and shape our lives in so many ways.

The power of "why" questions lies in the ability to get to the bottom of complex issues, and being able to fulfil a need that is required to fill.

How to find your Why

Short answer: you don't really have to.

As the short answer may not be exactly what you were looking for, let me elaborate further. You may have been born with your Why. Or you stumbled across your Why along the way.

The Why is your story.

The Why is such a compelling story, people are willing to sacrifice something about them to support your Why without being prompted. They don't act for the sake of rewards or incentives, but because they recognise a deeper meaning in their actions. Once again, it transcends from you in order to become theirs. That's why you should always make it your mission to find an audience who believe in your Why, and not rely on numbers.

75% of *highly influential people* agreed that sharing their message with others can have a true impact in the world around them. That feeling of overall fulfilment can be a key motivator for your Why.

Your Why is a great way to influence people by helping them reach a goal that they can relate to. By people connecting to your story, you'll be able to grow your influence. There is indeed a natural drive in people with a mutual goal, and often an influencer's job is simply to identify these group members and give them the best opportunity to reach that goal together.

Below there are my three favourite questions to define your Why:

- What is your mission?

- How do you want to help others?

- For what do you want to be remembered?

People buy into the passion, and passion comes from asking the right questions.

The right idea is not what drives your influence, your passion does - just like it did for the Wright brothers. When they built the first engine-powered plane in 1903, they had no team, finances or external support. Their motivation was making the impossible possible. That was their why - and their why gave them an advantage over their competitors.

A lot of marketers, scribbling away in their pads, or in an empty WordPress page, may disagree with that. To be incredibly frank, the Why may not be the direct answer to more sales, or more followers? As Simon Sinek mentioned in his 2009 TED Talk:

"People don't buy WHAT you do; they buy WHY you do it."[34]

That is undeniable. The Why will shape your figure as a leader, even if it's hard to quantify in terms of ROI (return on investment).

The best exercise from finding your Why comes from *Start with Why* by Simon Sinek, and it's linked to a very special Circle - a Golden one. The Golden Circle consists of three concentric circles with the "Why" as the main yolk, the "How" wrapped around like an egg white, and the "What" as the outermost circle.

Since the "What" is the easiest to know and articulate, most influencers start with the "What". We are human, and we do like to start on what we can control. So the idea is always more exciting, easier to define and execute. Sometimes they will also discuss "How", but they rarely talk about "Why".

You may be wondering the reason behind this. A lot of the time, the stronger the Why, the more painful it is. My Why is painfully vivid in my head, and when I am asked, I still struggle really going there.

As I mentioned in some of my stories so far, it's a mixture of very deep memories linked to my mental health, my loved ones and overall a very fragile time in my life.

I am always brought to tears when I think of it, and I can safely say there are a lot of things I still do not talk about as much. Your Why can be in itself a powerful exercise to uncover hidden feelings, fears and thoughts.

Is it worth it? Hell to the yeah.

Spending time refining your Why will help you with your setting individual goals, as well as telling compelling stories and going beyond fear.

The challenge of keeping your Why alive

As you may have gathered by now that the Why is no rocket science, the hardest thing after you find your Why is keeping it alive. *Highly influential people* agreed on this, with 75% of them acknowledging that sharing their message with others can have a true impact in the world around them.

The Why is a helpful reminder during the ups and the downs alike. Let's be honest, we all appreciate the power of motivation when times are tough, but why do we need to nurture our Why when things are blooming?

If the Why can help us snap right out of the hardship, it will be easily forgotten when short-term thinking and quick wins become more important, even though none of it reflects what your actual goals are.

It's a common sabotage of short-term gratification - which, to go all geeky on you Dear Reader, is very well linked to dopamine release[35] - a feeling that is also the reason why we spend more time on our phones than we probably do looking around us (thank you, WhatsApp group chats).

Just like notifications on your phones. Those opportunities that look appealing – but let's be honest, do not feel 100% right as well as the small victories and the new followers – become what we base our worth and overall achievements, rather than the age-old question: "Is this getting me closer to my Why?"

I am all for very straight-forward, no non-sense action steps.

Back in the day when audiotapes were a thing, Master Tony Robbins released the audio program of his *Unleash your Power within.* That tape truly changed my life, as it was the catalyst for me to leave my old job and start my solo career.

At the end of every single tape, he would remind me to take action. And I mean the end of every single one of them. You'd find me walking in the field, fist bumping the air, when Tony went "and now, it's time for you to take action". Seriously, right now, Tony?

Tony is not one for excuses, so you have to get it done. Most times I'd find myself scribbling down ideas on pieces of paper, or on my phone. You may find that a bit extreme, but the truth is, being able to channel our actions is what really keeps us strongly connected to our Why.

If you do follow the steps outlined in this book, and you consciously invest the time in getting back to your

Why, you'll find yourself less frazzled, demotivated and scattered.

Ultimately, the Why should be the basis for every decision you make and every message you pass along to others. Unsurprisingly, *highly influential people* agreed the reason they started their journey keeps them motivated when things get tough.

How your Why shapes your goals

*"The secret of getting ahead is getting started.
The secret of getting started is breaking your
complex, overwhelming tasks into small manageable
tasks, then starting on the first one."*

—MARK TWAIN

How can you use your Why proactively to drive you forward every day?

Your Why is, and should be, the solid foundation of your goals. Before you ask though, I am not going to have a lengthy monologue about goal setting - not that there's anything wrong with goal setting either – sparkling planners have their place (says the stationery addict).

However, there are a few ways you can truly tap into your goals in an effective way, and it comes down to mono-tasking and mono-goals. Numerous books, including *Single-tasking*[36] by as well numerous studies online have been suggesting it.

Still, I am the gal who likes her practical examples - welcome Joseph M Juran, and the Pareto Principle. Pareto Principle is named after an Italian economist, Vilfredo Pareto, who showed in his income distribution model that 80% of the land was owned by 20% of the people. Juran realised that this principle may, in fact, be a universal law: 80% of your results or outputs are always delivered by 20% of your work.

So less is more when it comes with goals, and our influencers prove this point. When asking our poll of influencers what is their main challenge when it comes to goals, 80% agreed that they don't know the steps to accomplish their big goals.

I always recommend setting one big goal, and a daily, small actionable goal you'll achieve before anything else.

Ask yourself: what am I going to achieve today to get one step closer to my Why?

Write down the whole list, then start prioritising. I am not here to tell you how to write your daily tasks, mainly as I am aware it differs from person to person. Just make sure your main action step is at the top, and that that one task is what you are going to prioritise for the day.

Coming back to the reward-triggered habits, ticking off lists does send a good message to our brain. So we tend to prioritise smaller tasks over longer ones. Please don't.

Write down the one task you'll get done first thing tomorrow, and give it your complete attention.

Goals are an essential motivator for you as much as they are for the people you are influencing. Rhiannon Lambert, the face behind *Rhitrition*, reiterated how her goal is fuelled by the drive of supporting as many people as possible, by providing the best tools according to people's needs: "*Motivation to help others (I hope my book can get to those who can't afford the help, this really drives me)*"

Your audience does and should come first.

Highly influential people agreed with the statement that they feel a "*deep emotional drive and commitment to succeeding, and it consistently forces me to work hard, stay disciplined, and push myself*". Let me ask you: can you recall a book you loved in which the main character just went about with no defined purpose or desire? Mostly not, and this is because a clear goal is vital to captivating an audience - and this is because of mirror neurons in our brains[37], the ones that make us perceive the actions as if it was us who was doing them. This is why, when sharing a goal for accountability to your tribe, you actually create a closer bond with them.

Try this simple exercise to really harness your goals: write one decision you've been putting off which, when you make them now, will change your life.

Now that you've made a real decision, you must take immediate action. To do that, write down the first few steps. What are three simple things you could do that would be consistent with your new goal? Who could you call? What could you commit to? What letter could you write? What could you do instead of your old behaviour?

My Why has changed. Now what?

All right, first and foremost do not panic. I knew you were going to ask - what can I say, I do know you, Dear Reader. We are human - ever changing and ever growing. So please, embrace the fact that your Why is going to evolve with you. Whether you are in your mission alone or with someone else, it's essential that you share your new Why with others - especially your tribe.

In June 2014, Jordan Younger broke the internet. Almost literally. On June 23rd, she published a blog post that took the health community by storm: "In the last few weeks, it's become clear to me how silly it is that I am so afraid to share this on the blog and in my life. It's not healthy to feel guilty for listening to your own body– I should be thanking myself, not telling myself I've done something wrong. I have *sinned.*"[38]

At the time Jordan was a very early "influencer": with over 300,000 followers, she was well on her way to celebrity-blogger status as a "wellness" expert and entrepreneur. Jordan Younger came out with her choice to move away from veganism and embrace a more balanced diet "I'm not writing about it because I think it's normal to share such personal aspects of one's life in such a public place... I actually think it's very abnormal, and it is counterintuitive for me to be doing this. I'm writing about it because I value you as my readers and friends tremendously, and I think it's time we ditch the labels".

Needless to say, the online reaction was huge and incredibly mixed: her blog crashed under the traffic, often made up of incredibly angry commenters. Nevertheless, she stuck to her guns, openly discussing her new lifestyle and new-found happiness. The episode culminated with Jordan's book *Breaking Vegan* a memoir about her journey through plant-based veganism, orthorexia and her overall relationship with food.

When sharing a mission to a broader audience online, you will be met with reservations along the way. If changing your opinion on high waist trousers may feel an incredible risk, admitting you are changing direction can feel incredibly daunting. However, it does showcase you, as someone willing to influence people are humble enough to admit things may have changed, and you are open to where your new why is going to take you. Some people like to write a long post, recording a video, write an email about what prompted you to this decision. Don't be afraid to go with your gut and adapt your Why to what is happening in your life.

It all comes back to the Why: Hazel Wallace, the Food Medic.

This lady needs no introduction whatsoever. What started as a working relationship, quickly turned into the most incredible friendship. I respect Hazel massively for her determination, work ethic and, obviously, her mission that clearly shines through in everything she does. We talked about her mission, the force behind the Food Medic, her upcoming plans and how she looked to disrupt the industry from within.

How did your experience as a young adult shape your decisions when it came to your future career?

When I was 14 years old, my father had a stroke at the dinner table. He was not an unhealthy man, but just before the stroke, he had been diagnosed with high blood pressure and type 2 diabetes. He was advised to watch his sugar intake and exercise regularly, and although I remember him checking his blood sugar every morning, I'm not sure how much nutritional advice he was ever given.

Losing him was the hardest experience that I have ever gone through. I will never fully get over the grief, but from his death, I have learnt a potent lesson. I have experienced first-hand how food can be a doubled edged sword - It can be the driver of disease, but it can also be a champion for good health. I guess that was the first seed to be sown regarding my interest between food and medicine. I decided I was going to be a doctor after we lost him, but it wasn't until I began blogging, while at medical school, that my passion for nutrition and lifestyle in the management and prevention of disease became truly evident.

Now as a doctor, it has become even more apparent to me that what we eat can have huge implications on our health, both positively and negatively. I come across lifestyle-related diseases such as type 2 diabetes, heart disease, stroke and dementia on a daily basis and I witness the frustration, from both patients and healthcare providers, at the dissatisfaction in the management of these conditions. There is a considerable disconnect between conventional medicine and nutrition, and that space has been primarily filled by unqualified opportunists, bloggers and pseudo-doctors who obscure any meaningful advances in understanding how nutrition influences health.

It's my mission to use my books, blogging and social media platforms to help manage (and prevent the development of lifestyle-related diseases by providing evidence-based advice on nutrition, physical activity, and stress management.

Why did you take a gap year from your job as a doctor, and how do you think is impacting your business with the Food Medic?

When you qualify as a doctor, you enter a 2-year foundation programme in the UK where you rotate between specialities. I decided to take a gap year between my first and second year, although I'm still working ad-hoc shifts at the hospital. I decided to take this gap year because I believe that I really have the opportunity to bring my brand to the next level and I couldn't simply offer it the time and energy it requires while training full time at the hospital. I also don't want my side business to impact my training as a doctor. It's all about finding balance. I hope to return to training at the end of the year and have a stronger business strategy (and team!) in place to assist this.

Why are you determined to still cultivate your career as a doctor, alongside your brand?

My dream was to become a doctor, not a blogger or an influencer - that happened by accident! But I realise that I am so incredibly lucky to have a platform to connect with people and share advice, recipes, and workouts to help people to live healthier and happier lives. I hope to progress my training and become a GP, but I would also love to continue working as a doctor online and hopefully on TV!

What's the main thing you are struggling with at the moment, and how are you looking to solve that?

I'm struggling to take the brand to the next level due to time, lack of experience and a lack of manpower! I plan to invest in business coaching and also in developing a team to work alongside me so that I can outsource some of the work which is holding me back from doing the things I really want to do.

What is your mission?

My mission is to provide incredible people with amazing tools to make a positive mark in the health and wellbeing of as many individuals as possible.

It's a goddamn heavy responsibility, but this is my calling. I could not see myself doing anything else. Truth is, the why is what everything always comes back to. I am here to show you the how.

I would love to share some of the incredible missions of some of the highly-influential people who joined my questionnaire. As you will notice, all of these people are on a mission of helping, empowering and supporting others. Can you see a thread there?

"To help the people around me accept themselves for who they are and understand that they can be whatever they want, life is a journey."

—CARLY ROWENA - PERSONAL TRAINER AND FITNESS BLOGGER

"To inspire a deeper global level of consciousness, shaping positive and sustainable change in health and happiness."

—CHELSEA PARSON - RECIPE CREATOR, FOOD INFLUENCER, CREATIVE CONTENT + PHOTOGRAPHER IN THE FOOD AND WELLNESS INDUSTRY

"To teach everyone how to live happier healthier lives"

—RUPY AUJLA - MEDICAL DOCTOR (MD).

"Inspire people to be more curious about who they are."

—CAT MEFFAN - YOGA TEACHER & BLOGGER

"I believe that health should not be a personal luxury, it should be a human right. My mission is to make it free and accessible."

—SHONA VERTUE - HEALTH AND FITNESS CONTENT CREATOR

"Inspire and influence women to stop doing what they hate, and start doing what they love. Travel more, work smarter, live happier."

—PHOEBE GREENACE - SILOU LONDON, YOGA TEACHER, TRAVEL BLOGGER, BUSINESS COACH

Habit Two: Diversify your Portfolio

Diversify, diversify, diversify... but first, focus

I am a book abuser. There, I said it.

Give me a paperback with any sort of relevant information, and I'll abuse it in a way bookworms would cringe about - or burn me at the stake, to use a much more vibrant analogy.

My book-abusing ritual includes the following:

- Highlighting
- Underscoring
- Annotations
- Exclamation marks

If a book receives the treatment mentioned above, it must be damn good. No surprise I had to literally bite my lower lip not to do the same with the *One Thing*[39] when it almost landed on my lap - actually, the Wi-Fi kept shoving it in my face. But hey, it wasn't my own copy. I have some sort of self- restraint. Occasionally.

However, it has been months since a book had me going nodding and clapping my hands - in that way only I seem to be able to pull off. The topic, needless to say, revolves around finding the one thing. "What's the ONE Thing you can do such that by doing it everything else will be easier or unnecessary?"

Man, that's a damn good question. In a world where our phones ping 24/7 and people are starving for attention, dedicating between three to four hours per day to one single thing sounds an abomination. Almost disgracefully indulgent. Seriously, do not tell me you have never gone on WhatsApp to check when your BFF, partner, or cousin had logged in last. Point proved.

Especially as one of the most infamous sayings of all times made its appearance in the book *don't put all of your eggs in one basket.* This is, quite unsurprisingly, an attitude we are used to in every single area of our lives. Whether it's boredom or fear of commitment, putting all our eggs in one basket is risky. Is it, really? Gary Keller surprises you with a front kick - can you tell I was a gamer in my past life?

The secret is to focus on growing one single area at a time, before focusing on new businesses or aspects of your business. I believe there is a place for diversification (so much so that we have a whole habit dedicated to it). However, diversification needs to come after you are clear on what you will focus your growth on first. I am the girl who moved to London and worked three jobs at the same time, after all. You cannot talk me out having different projects and passions, but I carefully choose what to focus on at any given time.

Different ways of growing your influence

"I've missed more than 9000 shots in my career. I've lost almost 300 games. Twenty-six times, I've been trusted to take the game-winning shot and missed. I've failed over and over and over again in my life."

—MICHEAL JORDAN

It's hard to admit you fail. Guess what: we all do - sometimes big time. Not too long ago I found myself in what some people may call *"the Divine Storm"* (the woo-lovers in the house will probably know what I am talking about).

For over 6 months as a company, we focused on mainly one product - and it came to bite us back in the bum - to be politically correct. I am talking stupidly high expenses, people needing to be fired in order to cut costs, and an overall personal and professional hell (which lasted overall about 4 months). The reason I am telling you this, Dear Reader, is because I felt lost. I felt like a failure (a topic that comes back again and again through this habit), but I also felt demoralised and started second-guessing everything I do, who I want to be, and what the company stands for. HBC was hit by a massive shit-storm (once again, keeping it classy Fab).

Without even realising, my survival instinct came in (something that you want to develop sooner rather than later). I knew that, unless I wanted to find myself homeless, penniless and soulless, I had to work my ass off and find other avenues. Now, I am not saying that everyone will experience this sort of *Divine Storm*. However, most of us do, from time to time.

The way I kept afloat and started re-building my business, strategy and overall life, was diversifying - and 93% of *highly influential people*, when asked about their income streams, agree they'd be looking to diversify streams of income by having different projects or jobs. What I always recommend clients I am mentoring is to find different areas and types of work that can secure different streams with different variables. Let me explain (yes, I am getting all geeky again).

Let's talk content first. I would always recommend building two to three media minimum, one of which must be your own (aka your website or email list). Others can be Instagram, YouTube, and Twitter etc. All of those who own everything you do, post or share. If you are not ready to sell yet, this is a way you can start diversifying from the get-go.

Content-avenues:

- Newsletter
- Website
- Blog

- Podcast

- YouTube

- Instagram

- Twitter

- Facebook

Same goes for streams of income. Do not be fooled: just because something worked for many years, it does not mean it will always do. Instead of breaking down every single service, I like to diversify income-avenues as follows:

- Seasonal Income

- Time-bound project

- Recurring Active Income

- Passive Income

- Recurring Passive Income

- One-off Fee

Now, because I feel I went deep down the rabbit hole of the business side of things, let me provide you with some examples for each one of those:

- Seasonal Income

  - Events

- Time-bound project

- o   Sponsored Post
- Recurring Active Income
  - o   Management / Monthly Content Creation
- Passive Income
  - o   EBook
- Recurring Passive Income
  - o   Membership
  - o   One-off Fee
- Speaking Fee

Since I literally split the company into two, I allowed us to diversify to diversify our offerings without adding more work and creating a base of recurring income, that can help when more significant time-bound projects may not be your primary support. Truth is, I used to be very vocal about putting all your eggs in one basket - however, as long as the basket is one, you can have different types of eggs to juggle with.

Why you should keep evolving?

Diversifying is key to thriving and being able to tackle what we perceive as failure. 95% of *highly influential people* agreed that they diversify their streams of income by having different projects/jobs.

One of the most incredible influential people I know – Rupy from the *Doctor's Kitchen* – is a doctor, a serial podcaster and author whilst also speaking at conferences and running his own online course. This allows him to spread his mission and touch as many people as possible.

It's evident that diversifying requires project management and organisation skills - nevertheless, I struggle to believe that most people were born with those. The essential skill to develop when diversifying what you offer and the topics you focus on, is to prioritise.

What is a priority anyway?

Depending on which definition you choose, there may be different nuances - however, this is by far my favourite:

> *"Something that is perceived as more important than other matters".* [40]

Perception is a big part of a priority, as it shapes the way we rank tasks, values, principles and projects in the first place. In Western societies, if a person is busy from having too much work, we assume they must be important. If a person isn't busy, they feel like they are not achieving enough. Welcome to the concept of urgency.

On top of our current programming, taking care of urgent responsibilities can give you an adrenaline rush, which makes you feel energised and alive. [41]

Instead of focusing on urgency, we should go back to (surprise, surprise) Habit One, which is closely linked to the overall mission and Why: having a clear vision for your future makes it easier to make choices and generally improve your overall management skills. Don't let urgency and to-do lists be what shapes your plans, but your mission.

An extreme and poignant example comes from Victor Frankl, a Holocaust survivor. He observed that the most common trait among the Holocaust survivors he knew wasn't their health, intelligence or family: it was their vision for the future.

"The lesson one could learn from Auschwitz and in other concentration camps, in the final analysis, was, those who were oriented toward a meaning (…) toward a meaning to be fulfilled by them in the future (…) were most likely to survive" beyond the experience. "The question was survival for what?"[42]

There is quite a powerful metaphor, linked to an experiment carried on by a professor, who once presented his students with an empty jar. He filled the jar with rocks and asked the students if they thought it was full. They said it was. In response, the professor poured in gravel, which filled in the gaps between the rocks. Next, he poured in sand, and finally, to completely fill even the tiniest gaps, he poured in water.

Think of that jar as the time in your life: the rocks as the important things, and the sand, gravel and water as the rest. If you put in the sand and gravel first – the unimportant daily chores – there won't be room left for the rocks. But when you put in the important things first, everything else will fall into place.

Questions to ask yourself before taking on a new project:

1. Is it in line with my overall mission and why?

2. Does it feel like a 'hell yeah'?

3. Is it going to support/help my audience?

If it ticks all the boxes, you are good to go.

On beating the failure ratio

Let's talk failure ratio. Don't look at me like that, Dear Reader. Trust me, failure ratio is a real thing: as real as unicorn lattes.

What failure ratio is, effectively, can be summarised as proactively deciding how many failures you are willing to accept before having a breakthrough. Some people have to fail six, seven, eight times to find that one thing that really works for them.

Failure sucks - massively. However, people will mostly remember your successes: behind every success, there's a list of failures, as each and every single one will take you closer to what you need to succeed.

Do you think it's just you and me?

Director Alfred Hitchcock shot the infamous shower scene in Psycho 78 times to get that moment just right. Let's be honest: the scene itself seems quite simple and straightforward. Nevertheless, to make it stick and become an icon of what tension is and has been in cinematic history, Alfred Hitchcock did not just settle for something that looked "okay".

As much as we can see this as sheer perfectionism, there is something about this example that also proves that most of what you do won't be perfect, great or even useful the first time you try it. Diversifying is what gives us space to play with what is not set, and keep going with what works.

How to diversify your brand with Phoebe Greenace

Silou was born in 2017 after I started consulting the founder Tatiana Kovylina on some logo, branding and marketing concepts, as my background is in marketing and start-ups. After a few months of working together, I took the role of CEO and co-founder as we complimented each other's skill sets and knew it was going to be a much bigger project than she first perceived. I had been blogging and creating my own personal brand for 5+ years at this stage, teaching yoga and also running a marketing consultancy so naturally all three business functions - product, service and content started to merge together.

How do you find the balance between running your content-based business and your product-based business?

Silou (www.siloulondon.com) takes up most of my time - I have a London based team plus freelancers in USA, Australia and remotely in the UK. My blog (woodandluxe.com) is a passion/hobby which leans itself to press trips, complimentary travel and brand collaborations which I do on the weekends and my free time. My service based business (teaching yoga) takes up about 5 hours per week. It's a delicate balance, but all of the businesses interlink and overlap and complement each other. The beauty in being the boss is that I'm not chained to a desk, so it makes having multiple focuses a little easier with freedom in my schedule.

What has been your most significant learning curve since starting Silou?

Producing an active wear line is no mean feat. It was more expensive than first expected, more time-consuming. There are huge learning curves in managing a production schedule as well as marketing, PR and design functions too. My background was not in fashion manufacturing, so I had to learn all of the things about seams, hems and fabrics. I've also had to learn to wear many hats in one day, and the learning never stops.

What do you think is the biggest misconception about having different streams of income?

I think it looks more glamorous than it is. It does look like I live the high life travelling to 5-star destinations with the blog, teaching yoga retreats abroad and hosting fashion campaign shoots. But the reality is, work never stops.

> *I struggle with my identity quite often. Am I a yoga teacher today? Am I a CEO bad-ass today? Am I a content creator?*

How do you make sure you take enough time to nurture both sides?

It's a delicate balance and not one I think I have entirely worked out. One thing that makes me stay sane is enough alone time and time on the yoga mat. If my self-care is taken care of, I am a more rounded human being. But saying that, I have overwhelming days too. No one is perfect. I am always evaluating if I still love everything I do and if it makes me happy. Maybe I won't have so many income streams in the future. Who knows!

How partnerships are shaping the way we influence

Like I mentioned a few times before, I am a self-proclaimed geek. Whether I am discussing lifting techniques or marketing practices, one of the things I enjoy the most is research (no wonder the preparation for this book literally felt like being a kid in a candy shop).

On top of general research and writing articles at the speed of light, I thoroughly enjoy writing reports and case studies. Every quarter we write a summary of the state of the health and wellness marketing industry - please do not roll your eyes just yet - and the beginning of 2018 became a fascinating time for influencers and brands.

Quoting our council member Emma Green from Bird & Bird, the way brands are viewing word of mouth has massively changed: "the wellness community is becoming more sophisticated and attractive to major brands looking to reach a new demographic, or stay relevant in the market. To achieve this, big brands may look at collaborating with a younger wellness influencer – these relationships should ideally be captured in a simple contract to make sure obligations and deliverables are clear, and both parties have clarity on how the relationship is intended to work."[43]

One of the most exciting aspects of creating content for others via your own channels has been revolving around content: "discussions over who owns content which is generated is also important, especially if one side is a blogger who wants to re-use content created under the relationship" continued Emma Green.

Are partnerships ESSENTIAL to be a successful influencer?

The short answer is No. However, collaboration can be an invaluable asset, not just for your wallet, but also for overall reputation and growth. This is why I always recommend a relationship over a transaction. Do not get me wrong, when a service is provided a transaction is expected - but how can you expect someone to know if you are the right fit if you do not get to truly understand them? I believe this is a conversation to be had with both companies and influencers, and only now the transparency is becoming the forefront of their relationships.

Overall, your relationship is closely linked to the people you align yourself with. When asking Hannah and Emily from *Twice the Health* about collaboration, they highlighted the importance of reputation: "We must BOTH be 100% in. If one has any doubts, we'll talk through these and will never go ahead unless completely happy. We will also only ever work with brands we believe in, and also believe are relevant to Twice the Health. No big figure will ever influence that."

When you have to sell yourself

Let's say you have set your boundaries concerning what you are going to align yourself with. How can you now evaluate opportunities worth your time?

When first getting started, a lot of influencers feel flattered at the idea of being approached to create content - the more the influence grows, the more dynamics seem to change. I am a firm believer in exchanges of values and long-term paid partnerships equally. However, it can take time to develop your boundaries, as well as your very own terms of how and when to accept certain types of work. I think Marisa from *Miss Marzipan* explains this quite effectively: "I won't accept an assignment that's clearly unbalanced in terms of reward. Case in point, a brand approached me offering $6 worth of spice mix in exchange for photography, recipe development, competition hosting via my channels and about two weeks' worth of work on my part. Yes, all for $6 of spice… which I already own. That's extreme, but there are loads of these "offers" that come my way."

Similarly, Niki from *Rebel Recipes* seems to echo Marisa when it comes to her decision-making process, involving "the correct ethos, a fair price, something I'm excited about". She also adds how "once working for yourself, you'll start feeling comfortable with the less busy periods.

There will always be ups and downs. Embrace the less busy times to take a step back and review where you are."

We need to bear in mind those discussions and negotiations are, objectively, what makes a business skill. There is this misconception that both parties are already experienced with how to handle any of these relationships by just having an Instagram account or a product to sell. This is not a way to discourage these kinds of conversations if anything it's to instil a certain level of confidence.

I have been talking about pricing methods and formulas more than what I'd have loved to. Mainly because, Dear Reader, the truth is, I do NOT have a fool-proof method. My gut tells me where to go, and it's quite easy. For example, if I feel physically sick when saying a price out loud, then that is not a sign of pushing myself out of my comfort zone but pushing my customers away because it may feel like I am uncomfortable with my worth. I know this is an incredibly tricky topic because you find people who will tell you "fake it until you make it" and "shoot for the stars". All I am saying to you is that I am NOT a salesperson, but I am selling all the time (and I love it too, just in case you are wondering if I am just incredibly masochistic). The reason I love it though is that I sell what I love, and I value myself enough to ask for money in exchange for what I offer people. As simple as that.

I remember when I first started my business and a "discovery call" was literally comparable to medieval torture. Now I meet, call, talk to people about what we do all the bloody time. Because I believe in the product, I believe in the people, AND in the audience I am talking to. Did this happen overnight? Absolutely not. I tried to get other people on it, I literally ran away from it as fast as I could because it felt somewhat unnatural. Guess what? Selling is not natural to most. However, if you want to work with people (and do not have an agent), you have to sell yourself. Thankfully by starting to sell yourself, you give enough value to what you do that you realise the worth of the time you spend helping others. If anything, this is such a crucial tool for your self-development (did I mention that embarking in this adventure is like a Tony Robbins seminar on steroids?)

Should I get an agent then?

This is another question I'd like to quickly address. You do not need an agent. Just like I did not need a salesperson to create opportunities. I think there is a place for an agent, but it is not for everyone. What are you looking to achieve? If you are in a place where you want to develop a personal brand around your lifestyle, your buying choices and partnership then yes, an agent could be an excellent way to go. However, the more you grow your influence, the more you'll have a clear idea of where you stand. Just like Hannah and Emily from *Twice the Health* explained, you'll be able to identify yourself when an opportunity is worth pursuing: "Always keep your morals in check. It's easy to get carried away with the campaign's objectives and beliefs and therefore sometimes lose sight of your own. Remember the content is to represent your brand, so this should always be at the forefront of your mind. Thankfully we have each other to keep in check, and ensure the content we create is balanced to both the brand we are working for and TTH."

How are you looking to develop your influence? How do you want to, objectively, change the world?

I know I am not the one for easy questions, but these are the questions that can help you find a direction in the way you want to make an impact. If you are still cringing at the idea of setting prices for yourself, we have tons of free resources to guide you with some pricing ideas. Will they be right ones for you? Unfortunately, I cannot ensure you that. My best bet is to ask: head to your community (just like the Health Bloggers Community) and ask others for advice and guidance - and, even if it feels so corny it hurts, let your instincts guide you.

You are your main product

For over 4 years, we have hosted HBCxMeet in around the country - that was, and still is one of our signature events. A mix of networking and educational talks, the meets have hosted incredible speakers who I admire and respect.

One of my favourite discussions must have been the one around self-love, mainly as it opened a candid discussion about boundaries and influence. Somebody from the audience asked *"What about the days I do not want to post content online? How can I meet those expectations?"* Our pretty unanimous response was "you should be allowed to cherish your time off" or "you do not really owe people to know if you are having a shit day". Nevertheless, most of us agreed we have all felt guilty/ lazy/anxious about not letting the world know about our bearings for 24 hours or more.

This opens up a much broader conversation about influence: in this 2.0 world, influence is pretty much married with information overload and a 24/7 reality. This translates with the apparent realisation that, when applying your influence into the outside world, we are all trying to make an impact. And that, my Dear Reader, requires a hell of a lot of work. When you are willing to influence people, you become your main product. The reason why I want to stress this - and I do believe I do not stress this enough - is because this means there should be boundaries, expectations should be set, and you should still have a degree of separation between you as a human and you as someone who creates content and harnesses influence.

Just like a domino effect, each habit follows the previous one - without really knowing who you are and what you stand for as an influencer, you will struggle to create a clear brand around you. *Highly influential people* agreed on the following: "I know who I am - I'm clear about my values, strengths, and weaknesses" while only 40% of *social influencers* say they are clear on their values and strengths.

Is your idea tattoo worthy?

During my long walk across town, (I love walking, it makes me feel like I am claiming my time back in such an easy way) I listened to a podcast episode with Seth Godin and Tim Ferris.[44] I typed down on my phone...

Is your idea tattoo worthy?

Whenever I get interviewed, every single interviewer asks me how I came up with the idea for Health Bloggers. All right, the stars did not align, I did not get hit by a lightning bolt with "*HBC*" on it (a bit like a twisted version of the Harry Potter origin story), , or woke up one day and knew it was going to work. I had no bloody clue. It just felt right at the time.

When I had to sacrifice my online coaching - all to protect my mental sanity, and fight my Virgo tendencies to overdo things - I did more or less what Seth talked about in the podcast episode.

The way for me to assess whether this idea that I was experimenting with was worth the risk, was to ask myself whether this community was one people would be proud to be a part of. Seth Godin makes an example with motorbikes, such as Harley Davidson and Suzuki. If you want to buy a motorbike, there are plenty of cheaper options than a Harley, but Harley comes with a message. An experience. A lifestyle. People do get a Harley Davidson tattoo, but certainly not a Suzuki one. Or Vespa - EEKS.

Of course, I am not suggesting you need to think whether your logo would be nicely wrapped around an arm of a 40-year-old trucker named Joe. However, I do believe that the people you genuinely want to help are the ones who can help you assess whether you are working towards a genius idea, or it's time to start over.

I definitely recommend checking this exercise from Seth's blog about something called *The First Ten*[45] - we get so excited about a new idea/ product/business, and we get so attached we are almost wary of asking our ideal market for opinions, in case they shrug their shoulders and walk away Beyoncé style.

Are only "new" ideas worth your time?

As I said before, and I shall say again, you do not have to reinvent the wheel. Use tools that already exist instead of struggling to come up with something completely ground-breaking. This is how Pinterest has become so successful. Pinterest simply repurposed the idea of the pin board and put it online so people could collect inspiring images and share them. This simple concept has allowed the site to experience a huge success.

Work and innovate when the time is right. When you need to devote yourself to your work, do it. Don't cut your work short, but also don't work when it's time for the other important things in your life, like family. Similarly, when you need to innovate, innovate. Don't innovate just for the sake of it –you'll only waste your creative energy. Save it for when it has the potential to lead to something great.

The sticky side of a personal brand

Coming back to the idea of being your own product, the real issues that come with being a personal brand is that liability and any legal ground are inevitably blurred. As part of our company, we also work as Whole Influence to create a robust set of regulations and legislation for marketers in the health and wellness industry.

From content ownership to collaborations, everything that is down to you using your influence goes way beyond your personal choice of a morning drink. Whatever you say online becomes liable to you as a personal brand, and this is one of the downsides of being your own product. This is also the reason why I always recommend our community and clients to really think about the conversations you are having online, as well as the way you engage with content.

As we go on discussing the role of a personal brand in the growth of your influence, we'll touch upon collaborations and partnerships and the way they are evolving within the online world. However, before thinking about partnerships, it's essential to create strong boundaries for yourself. I find there are a few ways that can really help you with creating more solid boundaries overall. You don't have to be your own brand: you can see the coaches, the nutritionists and the personal trainers shying away from creating a "brand", such as *The Food Medic* for example, and choose their name as a way to create some legacy that can be translated into speaking opportunities, books and other opportunities. However, most influencers who decide to use their own name as a vessel will also have some unrelated products or projects to support their own brand. Whether it's an entirely different company, or an extension of their current one (e.g. guides, products), it's a clear way to create a separation between the product and the person behind it.

Stand for something bigger: more and more influencers are launching their own campaign alongside their own mission, as a way to create an extra degree of separation, and also harness the power of community and collaboration. This can really help you reiterate your mission, as well as go beyond yourself to create a tighter relationship with your audience.

Emily is a gorgeous beam of light, keen yogi, mental health advocate and overall highly influential online figure. In 2017 she launched an online campaign to support the dialogue around mental health - we discuss how her TV experience helped her building her personal influence, as well as the learnings from her first campaign:

> *The exposure via Bravo is the reason that I have my audience so learning how to communicate over social media came hand in hand with building an audience.*

Launching a Campaign with Emily Warburton Adams

It has definitely made me more confident speaking over stories and I engage with some of my followers on a personal level because they have followed me from the very start while watching me on the show. While I have built a following post 'Below Deck', I am conscious of where my core following came from, which has meant that I keep my platform quite balanced and not explicitly focused on one thing. I have a designated "wellness"

Instagram page where it's all things health and fitness for the mind and body.

Growing my following after 'Below Deck' has enabled me to create an account that shares what I believe in more and more. I love this as I intend to share these messages and beliefs and (hopefully) be a positive influence. Those that have followed me from the start and have seen a change have either loved it and been great support or not liked it - but this is just life. On World Mental Health Day I ran this campaign to raise awareness around the topic and help break the stigma. It's an incredibly poignant topic for me as I suffered from mental illness for 6 years, spending time in and out of the hospital. When I left london, started work in yachting and later undertake the tv show. I redefined myself and the experiences I had, which helped me recover . Although I feel that if I had been honest about my medical history, I wouldn't have been granted that opportunity, and this is something that needs to change.

Campaigns like this are little steps in my journey to bring people together and create an impact. My long-term message is that people should feel able to speak out and that you can recover; that mental illness suffering and recovery makes you a stronger person through experience, and that action needs to be taken to help the prevention and treatment around mental illness. Social media is continuously transitioning, and we don't know where it will go with the content that's posted and how it's used. I shall say that I try to post with meaning and positivity, I attempt to be a good role model and influence for my followers. The platforms are sensitive so it can be hard to consistently do this but the feedback that I get motivates me, and it's very touching when people reach out and say that you've helped, or changed their mind-set for the day. The messages that I deliver are true to me and my core beliefs which I will start to push more and more. Mental Health and topics that people shy away from discussing openly are a niche, but I want to make this stand.

What it also comes down to is everyone is individual, different things work for us, and we have different intentions, so I always say that we have to be conscious of who we are following and how we use social media, as I'm not naive to its downsides. I plan to run further campaigns and associate myself with organisations and brands that share messages that align with my core belief and values.

Social media can be used to create positive and powerful initiatives, and I want to be a part of this and the stream of impactful social media use. Different, controversial content often gets the engagement and conversation, so I plan to share more original content that hopefully has this impact, along with the general posts, so I'm not pushing anything too heavy! I want to get followers involved in initiatives so that they feel a part of a community and movement as I believe we can have a positive power.

Drive for Daylight

After one of our events, I was walking back with one of our attendees: we were talking a bit about the company, goals, challenges, and hurdles. She looked at me, and she asked: "How does one manage to keep on going when things do not work out? You always seem to do so well." "A lot of the times thing do not go well. Being your own boss is like being on PMS every single day of the year." Probably one of my most quoted lines ever.

"What you can do, however, is let go of any idea as soon as it has gone out in the world. Simply put, you have no control of the outcome once it's out there. It's the nature of ideas in themselves." It can be incredibly frustrating at times, but it is the way you can sustain in business. You have to accept what does not work, and let it go if it's not working anymore. In the past 5 years, I launched over 10 courses.. One of them, probably my favourite, was a marketing course for yoga teachers (at a time when, sadly, the market was not ready). I launched my first (and only) round and had to accept it was just not going to fly. The idea and execution were excellent, but the timing was wrong. The purpose of focusing on the idea, not the outcome is at the base of what, in the incredible book *Creators Code46* they call *drive for daylight*.

Whether you are moving forwards or staying still, being clear about your values, strengths, and weaknesses is something 80% of our *highly influential people* have agreed on. I do believe that looking back to assess what did not work is essential to learn and grow, however, mulling over what did not work is what has a lot of businesses fail. When you are an influencer, and you are putting a lot of yourself into your work, driving for daylight is even more paramount: if something does not work, it is NOT a reflection on you.

Next time something does not work for you, this is what I'd recommend you focus on:

1. Keep track of your projects, and assess their overall performance. If something is not working anymore, ask yourself what has changed and assess whether it's time to adapt or let it go.

2. Once you decide to let go, give yourself some time to have a little wiggle, a cry or a tub of ice-cream (or even having a friend on call) and accept that it's time to move on.

3. What have you learnt from this experience: what will you repeat, and what should you not do again?

4. What's next for you? That, only the future will tell.

The attitude of focusing on the road ahead is what has stopped me from wasting time mulling over what did not work, and helped me take action to pro-actively solve problems and move past failed ideas.

My dear friend and influencer Chelsea founded *Well + Happy* around the time I started the HBC. It started as a popular blog and online resource, before evolving into chocolate. She is the prime example of how the feeling of "failure" is part of any given journey. This reflects the ways, as humans, we will be able to find what best works for us. When thinking about the way her business has changed she mentions: "We've now gone full circle right back to the foundations of the brand - food and positive vibes."

Coming full circle with Chelsea from "Well + Happy"

Well + Happy is now a wellness brand, designed to inspire a positive and purpose-filled lifestyle through food and affirmations, delivering this through an online magazine, events and retreats around the world. The brand educates and inspires others on the *Well + Happy* way of eating - fusing food, with positive vibes.

When recalling the old incarnation of the business, Chelsea admits that she had no idea of where it would take her: "I never intended on launching a chocolate brand, it just kind of happened. It took off and was so successful that I just kind of rolled with it - it was an incredible journey and experience, yet I reached a point where I realised that I just didn't want to be a chocolate manufacturer - so I stopped before I went too deep down the rabbit hole." Chelsea was feeling scared, anxious and uncertain. However, once she had made the decision it felt right, like a huge weight had been lifted. "I put a lot of pressure on myself to have all the answers and know what my next steps were going to be - but the transition time was so necessary for me to essentially grieve that part of my business and life" .If I had sat in a belief of failure, others would have felt it too. The grieve experience is undoubtedly the hardest part, when it comes to a failure: "even if it was the right thing to do, and you're excited by the change, when something is such a huge part of your life you will naturally go through a grief cycle, which you have to allow yourself to experience".

Whether we do agree with the idea that failure mainly comes down to semantics and much else, what society perceives as "failure" can be simply tackled as an idea that did not have the wings to fly. This is the reason why diversifying is key to being able to tap into your influence and truly make an impact: "I never really thought of my business closure as a failure, because staying in something that I didn't see myself growing with would have been more of a failure to me. I did, however, think others would think I was a failure, but again the whole process of grief and moving through it made me realise that the only way to move on and still ensure my brand was a success, was to show others that I was in that mind-set and energy."

One of the most important things when it comes to being able to go past the moments of grief is having a strong support network and the best tools to lift you up - I personally have a strong posse always around me to lift me up and send the odd GIF.

"My partner Jamie helped me realise the decision I needed to make without pushing me, yet supported me through the process. He's patiently listened to multiple business ideas, next step proposals, fears and wobbles - yet continues to motivate and encourage me to be the best version of myself."

Habit Three: How to Build Credibility in any Industry

The power of expertise

To better explain the power of expertise and how it indeed links to validation as a whole, I'll borrow an example from a bookstore. When people are out there, browsing for a specific book (in my case could be very likely an old classic or a cookbook), a few things tend to occur.

Let's use the cookbook example, as it feels much more relatable for most people. When spotting someone browsing in the food section, they'll mostly find first and foremost the cuisine / dietary lifestyle relevant to them. Secondly, they look at the author's name - as this will easily stand out instead of getting each and every single book out of the shelves for examination. Finally, the quality of the content will be the decisive fact. This theory was proven by a professor who, for the sake of experimenting, submitted a completely random article to a magazine; an article that did not make any sense at all. Despite the content itself, the article was published just because of his PhD. This gives people reassurance about the quality of the material, despite the actual content itself.[47]

A stellar 92% of *highly influential people* consider, as part of their mission, to *"educate as many people as possible"*. Not too surprisingly, even the *social influencers* seemed to agree with the statement, despite being much less suspicious than *highly influential people* when online personalities without any certification give questionable advice on the internet (a staggering 35% of social influencers versus 78% highly influential people) This clearly reflects the stance the general public has been taking recently when it comes to consuming content online, and shapes the way we approach information in a fast-moving world. However, don't be fooled by the idea that expertise is just a mere "trend" related to our sociological landscape. Expertise, to different extents, is part of the validation leaders have been harnessing for centuries before, making sure that also skills, charisma as well as creating a trustworthy image of themselves has been supporting their argument.

Indeed, you can fake it. So much so that an actor pretended to be a renowned professor and presented a talk for an audience of experts,[48] and purposely jeopardised it with repetitive and contradictory statements. By the end of the talk, the audience considered his talk highly informative. How did he manage to deceive a full panel of experts? He was faking, as well as acting: he appeared warm and friendly, sharing funny anecdotes while creating a charming yet fake professor character - this was enough to distract the audience.

This is not to wanting to put the seed of mistrust in you, Dear Reader. However, it comes to show that trustworthiness and expertise are not mutually exclusive, and perfectly work together.

Depending on what you want to specialise your influence, there are different avenues to boost your expertise. Most influencers I interviewed and who filled in our surveys have a certification of some kind and therefore tend to state that it's essential to have a certification to provide the best information possible.[49]

I am here to challenge this slightly - obviously. Despite the fact that degrees and PhDs are an incredible asset and should always be considered, I do believe there are so many ways to keep on learning (more on this in Habit Five).

- You can follow people with great influence and expertise

- You can listen to podcasts and watch TED talks

- You can read books, attend seminars and read studies

- You can write essays, studies and research

- You can embark on a new journey, such as a degree, course or study path

- You can network, by heading to a conference or a workshop

What you also should do is surround yourself with people that can complement your expertise. Let's be honest, we do not and should not be 360 experts in the subject that is life - once again, that would be stupendously impressive, but in that case, if not for my incredible wordplay, why would you be reading this book?

Most of us decide to focus on a specific area and in order to showcase expertise as well as inherent trustworthiness, having a solid network of people with better knowledge in some topics than you do is such a key aspect of harnessing your expertise - and recognising your own limits.

This is something industry standards, such as the ones created by a body like Wellspoken, address as content in or out of remit: if you are looking to discuss something outside of your area of expertise, providing recommendations that have been validated by a registered and credible professional or specialist is basically putting the consumer's safety and wellbeing first. Remember, in the health and wellness industry this is more important than ever - however, if your influence goes beyond that, you should be able to realise your limitations.

...and something more?

Lastly, though, if you are using your influence through the medium of content, you will have an added bonus - because you thought you'd be done, didn't you?

Content and the way content is presented are as important as your footnotes, especially as you do not want to alienate people who are coming to you with a problem to solve or an issue to resolve. I call this the "triple-whammy of credible influencers" (I know, I do have a talent for catchy names):

- Trustworthiness (how believable the content is)
- Clarity (how easily the content can be understood)
- Accuracy (how well documented the content is)

If you feel lost or overwhelmed, I recommend looking for codes of conduct and ethics within your niche and industry (I do recommend both the ones from theHealth Bloggers Community and Wellspoken Mark for health & wellness influencers). I am a very strong believer in the power of reliable content and continuous evolution through the medium of learning.

In the last 5 years, we have seen an incredible change in what is the way we consume, read and react to information. In a study from my buddies at *Wellspoken,* 73% of UK media reporting in general of the wellness industry and wellness brands, was negative in sentiment.[50] From the same study, we learnt that 74% of respondents identified that the least trustworthy wellness information was found on social media, shared by wellness brands and consumer health magazines.

Influencers are very aware of this as well, as in my study over 60% of them agree that they are likely to challenge people who give misleading information online.[51] It's a very important aspect of credibility, as it allows you to step back before producing any content or making any sort of judgement, and really think about what you are about to say. I want to highlight this because it's such a good practise to carry in your everyday life.

You know, the good old *think before you speak* habit we have been taught since very little. This also links back with another good catch-phrase *never argue when you are angry*. This is actually quite obvious, but so many of us do not seem to be able to follow it. The truth is, if you really want to showcase expertise in a professional manner, emotions cannot be what shapes your argument.

Emotions should be the fuel of any discussion (or piece of content, in this case), however, as soon as they take over what the rational argument appears to be, you quickly end up being in the wrong.

Who thought that learning how to harness your influence could also turn you into a better human? If you did not skip the first section, my Dear Reader, you'd know that influence is something that surrounds us on a daily basis, and we all influence so many people around us - from the Starbucks barista to the people following us online.

Being able to grow as individuals and shape our journey is what can also make us better influencers and help others getting there.

How can I make my content as credible as it can be?

There are so many ways to shape your content and make sure it's as credible and transparent as it can be (she says, with a bibliography as long as the Divine Comedy). Be excited about creating content you can learn from.

Challenge yourself by thinking about people you can tap into that can support you in areas you do not know, and find reliable resources for your articles and posts. Here I have listed my top five tips to make it easier for you to create credible content:

- Create a list of blogs, publications and websites to consult when discussing a very specific topic you want to support with further reading.

- If you have been taking a course or a degree, make sure you have saved the links to online resources and studies that your course provided you with - most courses and universities nowadays will have some to share with you.

- Take some time to choose how you are going to clearly list resources in your writing (May that be your articles or any online content). There is no right or wrong, just make sure people can clearly refer back to them.

- Build a list of contacts in topics and areas that are not your expertise, who are willing to help you out with quotes, articles or information when relevant.

By simply starting with these four tips and hacks, you'll be able to up your content game and save loads of time for yourself. By making it a habit, it will slowly become second nature to you - and reflect everything you talk about.

The power of language with Pixie Turner from Pixie Nutrition

If expertise and trustworthiness are essential, transparency in communication allows readers to check where your information comes from - something that in health and wellness is more important than ever. This is why I asked the lovely Pixie Turner - now published author of *The Wellness Rebel,* to answer a few questions about their message, information and content: "People out there are taking advantage of others' insecurities and fears, and exploiting them. We are seeing a rise in eating disorders and disordered eating, and these inaccurate and harmful messages are just fuelling the fire."

Why do you want to educate people to discern nutritional information?

There is so much misinformation on the internet, and we're all faced with information overload when it comes to nutrition and our health. I have personally felt the impact of that kind of misinformation spread on social media, and I want to prevent that from happening to others, so I speak out against the BS I see and hope it helps! It's also a great way for me to vent my anger and frustration in a way that's both therapeutic and hopefully entertaining!

How do you think this can help people on a wider scale?

On a simple level, I hope it saves someone from spending unnecessary money on products they don't need. On a deeper level, I'm hoping that it'll empower people to appreciate the complexities of nutrition, develop a greater understanding of the scientific method, and improve their critical thinking skills.

How do you make sure you support your audience in the best way possible when it comes to content and research?

My tactic on Instagram is to draw people in with the pretty food pictures, and then throw some science at them. If I'm writing about a topic that I'm not 100% sure about, whether it's in a blog post or an Instagram caption, I'll get someone to check it over for me and make sure it's all correct. I'm also very careful about my wording and phrasing on social media; I take great care to ensure I don't use triggering language and always try to attack ideas rather than the person. What I don't want is for people to feel like I'm being condescending or making fun of them for falling for pseudoscience.

How do you make sure you are always up to date when it comes to studies, trends and fads?

As a nutritionist registered with the Association for Nutrition, I have to make sure I undergo continuous professional development in order to stay on the register. That can be in the form of courses, conferences, and so on. I also have conversations with nutritionists, dietitians, and researchers both in person and on Twitter. Trends and fads I tend to spot on social media, and often react immediately to things I see on there.

Where do you think language fits into this conversation?

The language we use to talk about food really matters. It affects the way we perceive food and ourselves. Using morally charged, triggering, or fear-mongering language can lead to disordered relationships with food.

What makes something credible?

If defining what makes influence was no mean feat, finding *what* makes something or someone credible was even harder. I do believe this comes down mainly to the fact that credibility is a word that has been associated with leadership as much as it has been associated with expertise.

I personally believe that not all experts are leaders, but leaders should all be experts. This is where the proverbial cookie crumbles; on top of this cookie (which I like to imagine as being a chocolate chip one) you'll find both objective and subjective components of the believability of people themselves.

Key components of credibility are trustworthiness and expertise, with other ingredients including measurements and reliability (what you could call "track record"). Experts really add an extra layer to the credibility formula, including ingredients such as credentials, certification or information quality.[52] This is where being an expert has felt like, namely, *shitloads* of work.

The theory of the "10,000-hour rule" by psychologist K. Anders Ericsson states that it takes 10,000 hours to become an expert in a field. Author Malcolm Gladwell brought the idea into the mainstream in his book *Outliers*, still highlighting the importance of ability as well as time to develop a skill. The theory has now been refuted and questioned; however, it's undeniable that time is an essential aspect when developing expertise.

When it comes to credibility, it's essential to always remember the importance of storytelling: keep things enticing enough for your audience, for them to be willing to listen to what you have to say.

I know, I am the first one to admit I can be extremely verbose and spend hours dwelling into a specific topic just because I become genuinely obsessed with a specific issue or problem. Although it's known that detailed information is important for credibility, no one likes to be bombarded with too much information. As humans - funny little ones we are - we tend to shy away from too many options, but we do like to have options: just like the Goldilocks principle[53], a few options will give us a choice, too many will make us lose our interest in the task at hand.

Now that we can see all the ingredients for credibility, it's essential to look at its foundations: trustworthiness and expertise separately.

Trustworthiness.

My dear friend and side-hustle partner Sarah Greenidge from *Wellspoken Mark* is a bastion of credibility. In our joint training scheme, we clearly highlight the importance of providing the best information in order to create a trustworthy relationship with your audience. Just like any kind of relationship, a relationship with an audience has to be based on a level of respect and overall transparency.

The truth about trustworthiness is that it can easily compensate for lack of expertise, especially as, for example, influencers are embarking on a journey to undertake a new career or enrol to a course etc. Despite not being the no.1 fan of buzzwords, the idea of post-truth sums up what our society has shaped up to be from the early 2000s onwards.

Post-truth was The Oxford dictionaries Word of the year for 2016 and was defined as "an adjective defined as relating to or denoting circumstances in which objective facts are less influential in shaping public opinion than appeals to emotion and personal belief".[54]

Aside from being undoubtedly frustrating to some extents, post-truth does reflect how much emotions and personal beliefs affect the world around us - yes, Tony Robbin was right all along.

Jokes aside, trustworthiness is the foundation as much as expertise makes the bricks of the house. Let's put it this way: you may have all the certifications and degrees in the world, but if you are not able to put your audience in a position of transparency and security about the information you provide, you only create confusion and mistrust, and your influence is tainted.

As well as post-truth, another trait that can steer us in the wrong direction when it comes to trustworthiness is our tendency to only seek out and pay attention to information that agrees with what we already believe: this is known as confirmation bias.[55]

Confirmation bias is also something that leaders, in some respect, will harness in order to create a sense of belonging among people around them. Tapping into emotions is powerful: when people are emotionally invested, they join movements, buy products and brands – and even use them as symbols to show others who they are and who they support.

The trust people put in you, becomes something they can proudly show and ultimately tells their audience, friends and peers something about them. Once again, confirming their own emotions and beliefs.

If this seems quite daunting as a window in the human psyche, it's important to remember that this is just how we act and behave as humans. The fact that our online world has amplified that, does not necessarily change the fact it been a need we have always had in the first place. However, just like with Peter Parker and his "with great power comes great responsibility", the difference can be made when we use these techniques to create a safe environment for our audience.

I remember while studying for my PT exam, I realised that learning about a new tool, or a new practical skill in a matter of hours confused the hell out of me.

Nevertheless, I knew that to be a good personal trainer I wanted to be able to answer any Why that may come my way within my area of remit (while trying not to get too geeky and show clients infographics squats), and this is why I spent hours looking at veins, arteries and lungs.

When I later started working with clients, what I realised was that being able to quote my sources, as much as accepting my limitations made my clients feel more secure - and kept the bullshit factor to something pretty much close to zero.

I also believe that depending on *how* and *what* you want to influence people on, the way you communicate certain information will be different - and the references, as well as sources will be cited differently. Plus, you are entitled to have opinions, and this is incredibly important as well.

Nevertheless, *because* of your influence, you owe your audience the transparency that allows them to look into any bold statement you may make (guess what, you are allowed those!) which also leads me to a VIP (very important passage): learn how to read your sources.

As Rhiannon from *Rhitrition* also pointed out to me when discussing credibility, the impact you'll have will be placed on real people "I see the destructive impact ill-informed advice can have of an individual's health on a daily basis in my clinic. Poor advice can affect mental and physical health long term. I work with eating disorders, and this has enhanced my drive to do something about this."

I work with influencers and bloggers in health and wellness, and thankfully I have a good understanding of how to read some studies, and how to interpret and re-share some of the findings. Sometimes, just like the old PT days, I still have to read the same passage thirty times before it sinks in. However, I believe spending the time (or investing in some training) on how to read and present a study can be essential for some people who are still looking to develop specific expertise.

What happens when you break someone's trust?

A few years ago, back in my coaching days, I would organise quite a few webinars for my audience. There was a particular instance when everything that could have gone wrong did.

On that day a few key things happened:

- On the same morning, my internet connection disappeared.

- My webinar hosting service decided it wasn't a good idea to record the class.

- I mistakenly uploaded the video on the wrong YouTube channel.

- I had problems with embedding the YouTube video.

This is a mere example of how, sometimes, things can just go wrong. Whether it's beyond your control, or you somehow did break someone's trust, it's important to own whatever happens.

There are so many ways we can mess up things in life: that link leads to a 404, the password is not working, and the eBook you received is in Hungarian?

It's very simple for people to avoid confrontation, and therefore avoid rectifying a situation: rather than moaning and just binning an unsolicited email, you can take action about a situation you are not happy with by letting people know.

So many people just shrug shoulders, get irritated and move on, but would that change the situation in any way? Would that fix the link, or your email magically unsubscribe out of rage?

My best advice is always the same, regardless: be honest, be transparent, and let people know what's going on. Rather than frantically trying to fix the matter as soon as possible, give people a heads up, and take your time in order to ensure you know what happened and what you are looking to fix.

I am Italian, so this comes without saying for me: if there is a problem, not only I fix it, but I thank people for being understanding - and occasionally bring homemade food to make up for it.

It's just the way I am. Anything extra you can give people to show that you understand the frustration, and are willing to make up for that; you are, quite frankly, just letting them know you are there for them.

Accept that you can and will make mistakes in the most humble possible way.

Rather than hitting yourself up learn from your mistakes and be sure it doesn't happen again. The most obvious way to avoid a breach of trust is to be aware and prepared.

New problems will arise, but you will have a bulletproof strategy to fix them in the most loving way possible. Whatever the situation may be, in life rarely things go to plan: recognise when and how you were wrong, and actively try to make up for that with your actions and gestures - whether it's rectifying an old statement, editing a blog post, or privately apologising for an inappropriate comment. Being able to admit your own faults is also what builds on credibility.

What's the evidence in wellness? With Kimberley Wilson

It was a pleasure and honour to have Kimberley answer some questions for me on the topic of evidence, wellness and credibility. Kimberley is very vocal on the topic, and her event was a response to this - hence me asking her to be involved with this project.

Could you please share a bit more about "Wellness: what's the evidence?" and why you decided to run this event?

The conference was born out of a few things. First, was a worry about what I saw in my psychology practice. Many of the people I work with have issues with eating, whether they have been diagnosed with eating disorders or have more generalised disordered eating behaviours. My clients were reporting their inaccurate beliefs about food, particular nutrients or special diets that, from my qualification in nutrition, I knew to be untrue. But because they had read them several times on influential social media accounts, they were convinced that the information was accurate. I realised that inaccurate health information on social media was really harming people and reducing their likelihood of recovery.

Secondly, I became frustrated that there were many unqualified people setting themselves up (sometimes unintentionally) as health or nutrition experts. I don't think many influencers truly appreciate the power that they wield over their audiences or desperate people who are looking for answers.

The conference was my response to these observations and concerns.

I knew there were qualified experts out there each doing great things in their corners of social media and I thought it would be valuable to bring these people, who I respect so much, together in one central point so that we could offer a unified voice on what the actual evidence says and give attendees the opportunity to ask questions directly.

What was the biggest takeaway point?

There were a few. One thing that I realised was that there is a lot of confusion out there around health, wellness and nutrition. People are really confused about what to do, and this makes anyone who is offering a simple-sounding solution more attractive. In reality, nothing is really that simple, and experts need to work very hard to convey that message and make it one that people want to listen to.

Another major issue that was raised by the audience was their concern for young people. The messages about health, beauty and success that are so common on social media are creating huge pressure for young people. Parents were particularly concerned that their children are constantly exposed to potentially damaging messages, and they cannot always be there to supervise or rationalise what they are reading. It is a concern that I share. Most social media platforms are only 10-15 years old, and we don't fully know the impact they might have on young minds, though there is early research that indicates that excessive use is linked with increased anxiety and depression.

Most studies and research seem to agree that credibility is mainly made of trustworthiness and expertise: do you think there is anything else we may be forgetting in this formula?

I think in the past truthfulness and expertise may have been sufficient, but I believe that the landscape is changing. The internet and social media have democratised information, which in one sense is great; more people have access to information than ever before. However, the downside is that anyone can set themselves up as an expert and build an audience with content that might be, at best useless or, at worst, actively dangerous.

I think, in the future, credibility will also involve an aspect of popularity; the number of followers or endorsements by other influential people or institutions. The challenge for experts and researchers is to be able to present their information in an attractive way that is appealing on new media platforms. Old school authority just won't be enough.

Do you think confirmation bias affects the way we perceive information online, and if so, how?

I'm sure it must. In general, we like to feel consistent with our beliefs, so we tend to seek out information that confirms what we already believe. On top of that the brain processes information that confirms our pre-existing beliefs as 'facts' compared to information that contradicts it. Finally, sometimes the facts don't even matter. We are deeply influenced by the way in which information is conveyed, so we are more likely to believe or agree with something said by someone we admire or aspire to be like than someone we do not (this is the power of celebrity endorsements). Putting that all together, it takes a lot of work to change your mind on something even if the evidence itself is compelling.

Why do you think there is a lot of mistrust in health and wellness?

As I mentioned, the democratisation of information has created a lot of 'experts', some qualified, some 'qualified by experience', some completely unqualified. But if all of these people are convincing in the way make their cases (especially if they believe it themselves) it can be very difficult to distinguish whose message is the most accurate and useful.

It's also true that some aspects of the media do not help. The shift from print to digital media has meant that there is much more competition for readers. In order to compete, editors have to create compelling, sensationalised or alarming headlines. This means that even well-conducted research can be distorted in the drive for clicks. And then comes the inevitable rebuttal ('that's not what it means') and you can understand why readers are confused or distrusting.

How do you think personal education and being able to spot myths is important to build credibility and trust in the industry?

I think, in order to keep themselves safe, audiences are going to have to develop a lot more scepticism when viewing information online, and take less of it at face value. Ask content creators for their credentials. Are they working within their area of expertise? What do their critics have to say? Do they engage honestly with criticism or are they involved in personal attacks? My experience is that, when it is not about ego, people are happy to engage with questions. When it's about ego people, become vague, defensive and hostile.

There is an important role in helping people to spot the signs of nonsense compared to good information. Hopefully, we'll start to see more of these types of tools.

How would you rectify in the case of you breaching your audience's trust?

Just be honest. If you have made a genuine mistake; explain, as best you can, what happened, apologise and commit to being more judicious in the future. In most cases audiences respond really well to this; it shows that the content creator is human and has enough personal integrity and respect for their audience, to tell the truth.

It's more difficult where there has been actual deception - for example saying your weight loss results were due to an exercise routine you're promoting when in fact you went on a secret crash diet. I think this sort of thing is really disrespectful and the audience can end up feeling used; the creator doesn't really care about them they just want to make money. In this case, an apology is also essential and perhaps a personal commitment to be more respectful of the trust that their audience puts in them.

Habit Four:
The Power of
Community

What is a community, anyway?

"The secret of leadership is simple: Do what you believe in. Paint a picture of the future. Go there. People will follow."

—SETH GODIN, TRIBES

When looking at the definition of community in any dictionary, the constant buzzwords come up; common interests, common attitude, commonplace of living etc...

However, personally, I believe that a community is much more than these things. The best definition of what I see a community as comes from Seth Godin's *Tribe*, and it includes building blocks such as; a group of people, shared cause, a leader and a story[56] (yes, Habit One is back to bite you right in the bum - oh, did I forget to mention to you that these habits are all correlated?)

To build a community you need a Why, a clear mission linked to a story and to share your Why and story, you need to have a community around you. Whether you create your own or you find one - this is a topic we'll discuss later in this section.

Community has always been with us, but with technology, the number of communities cropping up is exploding. It's important to realise that you do not need to create a Facebook group, a series of events, a forum or an elaborate website to give your community the space to grow.

However, a community is something powerful and is what you need to grow your influence. Remember, 9 times out of 10 people will come to you organically, all you need is a place for them to interact, discuss and grow.

Social media (and the wonders of the online world) has allowed something different to happen since the times when communities were gathering in a physical space. It has moved the communication from vertical, as in between you, the leader, and the individual members, into horizontal communication, as in communication between members.

Once you see how you are facilitating a conversation between others, you quickly realise that the community is as much about you as it is about people who make the community itself. Furthermore, it is about the relationships between your members.

This is where social media has allowed us to really come together and facilitate introductions by facilitating collaborations between others.

Starting vs finding a community

I do find that most people tend to find a community to belong to before starting their own. Some people get so invested into the community they join they may decide to support it actively by representing it (just like our ambassadors).

Your website, blogs and social media accounts are not just there for you to share stories but also to provide the room (and the tools) for the community to communicate, share ideas and network. How actively you manage and coordinate that, is objectively up to you, and will not necessarily impact in the way the community grows.

Let's say you are not interested in hosting meetups or creating a private group of people to discuss a specific topic. There are so many other ways you can facilitate community interaction. Here are a few examples;

- Twitter Chats
- Instagram Live
- Webinar
- Facebook Live
- Collaborative Articles
- Interviews
- Speaking at an Event

A lot of these examples do facilitate conversation and growth by allowing people to actively interact with you and other people. You can bring members closer together by facilitating communication and tightening their common bonds. You can do this by transforming a shared interest into one passionate goal, and by providing a platform for members to easily connect with each other.

Once again, not rocket science; just the way the online world is shaping itself.

By finding a bigger community, you can start a conversation with the people who follow you and ask them to put forward how they'd like to interact with you, either online or offline. In the meantime, learning from other members of that existing community as well as finding new people to connect with.

I am a believer that to start your own community you need to find other communities that you are willing to belong to and participate in.

How many people do we need to start a community?

This is not an exact science; however, Kevin Kelly author of the famous article, 1,000 True Fans[57] says that a true fan happens to be a member of the community who cares deeply about you and your work.[58] These are the customers that will repeatedly buy from you, the followers that will interact with your content, the audience taking action every time you ask them to.

I can hear you saying, wrinkling your nose and narrowing your eyes: "1,000? Is this enough Fab?" In a world where millions of people can read your captions, like your pictures and watch your daily life broadcasted online, are we sure 1,000 is still a relevant number? The answer is yes, 1,000 is all you need.

This is the number of people you need to support you to make a living, to reach more people, to be better. It's enough because this is what you need to create a community. That bold and beautiful Why that you shaped, let it be what drives your tribe to higher heights: it shapes your community values and ideas allowing others to relate to them and wanting to spread them.

Remember when we discussed, back in Habit Two about your ideas being 'tattoo-worthy'? I used the example of Harley Davidson and how the company has built up a massive community of loyal followers over the course of their 100-year existence. This is precisely what I mean when I talk about your Why shaping the community.

For its customers, a Harley isn't just a motorcycle, but a symbol so crucial to them that they're willing to wait several months for a bike they've ordered – and, in the meantime, get the company's logo tattooed on their arms.[59]

A strong Why simply allows people to be directly engaged in the movement by scratching an itch that hasn't been sufficiently scratched yet? This is what turn members of a community into driven believers instead of just followers - and has them beat the social media drum for you. A great example of a community is CrossFit.

It all started in 1995. Greg Glassman, now known as "the Coach" established a gym in Santa Cruz, while also training the Santa Cruz Police Department.

As the work began to pile up, he decided to introduce group sessions, finding out that he could still offer enough individual attention to each client to ensure safe and effective training. He then started a website where fitness lovers could connect and exchange programs and advice, as well as follow the joint program devised by Glassman. This was a way for Glassman to give back to the community. He understood how to lead a community by telling stories and giving people the possibility to connect together via the website.

CrossFit was formally established in 2000. The company's first affiliate was CrossFit North in Seattle. By 2005, there were 13 affiliates. By 2012 there were. 3,400 affiliates worldwide. CrossFit certification courses are now available worldwide, and CrossFit gyms are opening up all over. The annual CrossFit Games are now broadcasted worldwide, and thousands of athletes compete for the title of 'The Fittest of Earth'.

To recap, what are the building blocks of a community, the ones that you should have to nurture your very own?

- A leader (that's you, that is)

- A strong message to share

- A group of people to share this message to

Are you ready to be a leader?

In Habit One we talked about fear, discomfort and pushing boundaries. A leader steps right into this discomfort zone and gets organised so that people will follow them.

It's interesting how we have this idea of leaders as people who lead. It's in the word itself, and therefore they are somewhat looked up to.

The best leaders are actually the ones able to begin movements by empowering the members of their community to communicate. They are the ones establishing the foundation for people to make connections, as opposed to commanding people to follow them.

Nevertheless, we are taught that people buy into an idea. I'd like to challenge that by actually saying that, in fairness, people buy from people.

Disclaimer: this was something my dear friend Vicky told me once over the phone, and clearly stuck with me.

Coming back to our building blocks of creating a community, there are three things leaders can actively do to nurture their community:

- Take the shared passion and mission and turn into actionable goals for the community

- Leverage current members to grow and expand the impact of the community

- Provide tools and ways to allow members to communicate and collaborate

By leading, you are essentially creating something worth talking about (just like you would do with your message). The community itself becomes a product of your influence and as word-of-mouth grows its relevance is as much as your mission as anything else.

People in leadership positions who want to get others to take action always begin by explaining why something has to be done. That way, they create a sense of belonging which makes others take action.

This is where peer pressure comes in. In addition to strong ties such as close friends, social spheres the online world is made out of acquaintances, especially thanks to the way we feel like we do end up knowing people we can only see through a screen.

People often ask me how sharing your life online can attract so many people - regardless of how well they know you. This is because your close friends are not the most powerful advocates. It is mostly via less strong ties that peer pressure is exerted. When a person's friends and acquaintances support an idea or a mission, it is hard to opt out.[60] In the same way, when someone you admire is part of a community, you are more likely to be wanting to join it.

To lead, you must be able to inspire action within a community.

The way people tend to be within a certain environment is inherently passive, but occasionally, we do feel prompted to be active in our behaviours.

By being the good leader of a community, you'll be the one inspiring the action you want people to take in order to grow within the community. From moderating communication to inspiring debate, a good leader is the one who is a champion of accountability and inspiration.

This also means that being a leader is a lot of work. It's also important to remember that, depending on the kind of community you are gathering, it's hard to micro-manage the members that will be joining the community.

How should you run your community?

Leaders in the workplace are incredibly aware of the people they bring in to their space. The book The Ideal Team Player by Patrick Lecioni clearly outlines some great characteristics of team players who can positively affect the team on the whole. Aspects of good team players include

1. Hunger to go above and beyond.

2. The social smarts to interact positively with a group.

3. The humility to let go of your ego for the team's common good.[61]

When looking to scale a larger community, it's hard to veto every single member on the basis of those aspects. However, I always recommend finding a select number of members who you think can bring those traits to the community at large.

These are going to be your ambassadors, your vocal advocates.

In an ideal scenario, the community's goals will transcend from each member's personal success, to make sure the overall team is happy, functional and supportive. Once again, something that sounds so simple and obvious, but it makes such a difference in the way the community is run. Reminding your community of the bigger picture and the Why will make them truly invested in what the community stands for.

When talking about the concept of dysfunctional teams, Patrick Lecioni[62] highlights some key traits that can disrupt the overall harmony of the team. Lacking accountability is one of them: and it's not just the accountability we discussed before, but also the inability of calling individual members out for mistakes, or the lack of trust in the community itself and its ability to support the members towards the main goal.

By creating a safe environment that encourages healthy debate and questioning, the community will be able to take collective decisions to facilitate the growth of the community as a whole. When looking at asking for help and support from the community to facilitate growth and expansion, I always recommend coming back to those selected members, those ambassadors that are active, engaged, and clearly represent the community as a whole.

Ideal ambassadors are humble: a humble person will be quick to point out the contributions that other members make and define success collectively, strengthening the community feeling. Ideal ambassadors are also hungry; these people are always in search of more: more achievement, more learning and more responsibility. These types of people do way more than what is expected because they're driven and passionate about the community and the message behind it.

The truth is, the leader's role as a facilitator allows the community to run itself and foster new leaders in the making. It's a beautiful cycle that is almost as rewarding as the creation of the community itself.

The power of engaging in a community

"Tell a story to people who want to hear it. Help them connect as a tribe. Lead the movement. And finally, make a change."

—SETH GODIN - TRIBES

People have the misconception that game-changing-ideas have to be grandiose (and preferably supported by elaborated stunts and a cinematic soundtrack).

This is not true.

The Health Bloggers Community was actually born on a rather wet afternoon nearby Victoria station in London. I was meeting an online friend for the first time, and at the time I was a 24-year-old with a lot of dreams and a very confused plan (not to mention that I had no idea of what the future was holding for me - ah, Universe, you funny thing).

My friend told me about a place that did smoothies and juices (such a novelty in London at the time), so we gladly went through the back alleys to find this hidden gem. We were chatting about her plans to leave her job and become a full-time yoga teacher. I was telling her how green juices changed my life (that transitional moment in my life where green juice was a novelty).

As we walked back, I vividly remember us sharing frustrations about how none of our friends would understand our passion for crystals and meditation. Most of my friends would likely not show up to morning yoga classes, as they were recovering from royal hangovers on a Sunday morning.

"I wish there were a group where people could talk about their passion for health," she said.

That's what I am going to do! I immediately thought to myself, and my face visibly lit up.

"Leave that with me" I replied.

And Ta-Dah. A week later I had a name: "Health Bloggers UK". I started a Facebook group and a weekly Twitter chat - which loads of people do still remember fondly. As the group grew in size and relevance, I decided to evolve my idea (a hobby that was taking about 10 to 15 hours per week).

Shortly afterwards, I changed the name to the Health Bloggers Community or HBC. Admittedly, I find this to be the most self-referencing name in the history of brand names. If you have a health blog, then you need to come to the Health Bloggers Community. Simple.

The HBC went from being a community to being an educational resource, a platform of growth and the main body of authority for bloggers and influencers. We host a Summit, an Awards Ceremony and so much more. The community itself is a living and breathing organism, where everyone is willing to help, support and provide encouragement.

I believe that the beauty of the HBC stands in the way we encourage collaboration and conversation, and how this turned it into an invaluable resource for bloggers. The team is just the glue that holds the vision together, but the members are what truly makes it.

I cannot stress it enough - being a passive member of a community is not conducive to growth. Being open to discussion, collaboration and offering your expertise is what will grow your influence beyond any stretch of the imagination. The easiest thing is to react. The second easiest thing is to respond. But the hardest thing is to initiate.[63] By inspiring others, we establish a following.

As mentioned before, just like with the matter of influence, it does not matter who these people are. Whether they're your audience, customers, or employees, excited followers are the most loyal. And, backed by them, we can change an entire industry - or, if we want to be bold, the world.

How collaborating can support your growth

The below examples are not just an exercise in self-indulgence, but a small sample of how my community has responded positively to how I have implemented the habits highlighted in this book. It is a progressive movement to allow the community to share big changes and steps they have taken since joining and is a way to clearly see that the impact you have (as the group leader) goes beyond what you may see on a daily basis.

"The Health bloggers community portal is packed full of amazing tools, tips, valuable, practical, useable information and knowledge. It's a real community of support, collaboration and accountability to grow goodness together. I've been blogging and coaching in the wellness industry for over 20 years and feel it's an invaluable resource for everyone, whatever stage you are at. I would highly recommend joining."

—KIM MULTI AWARD WINNING MIND BODY NINJA, AUTHOR AND TEDX

"Through HBC I've met some wonderful people. Like-minded people who now inspire me every day with the work they do. Although I've only been a HBC-er for a few months, my skills and confidence have grown. This growth I attribute to the close-knit nature of the group and the undying support we all show each other."

—AMY MEEGAN, THE BAKING NUTRITIONIST

"The HBC has been incredible for me - not only in my blogging journey, but also life in general as I have met the most inspiring & supportive people through this community!"

—ROMY, ROMY LONDON UK

"I love being part of the Health Bloggers Community. It really does live up to its name; I've met so many friends through the community and there is a real spirit of support and collaboration. I feel that being part of the HBC has increased my confidence in my blog and given me many new opportunities."

—RACHEL EVANS, HEALTHY AND PSYCHED

"I've been a part of the HBC community for what feels partly like a short time and partly like a long time. Short because I think it's only been three months. Long because so much has changed and evolved since being welcomed into the community so greatly. HBC has given me the chance to attend the summit and learn from other blogger & influencers. It's also given me the opportunity to grow and create events in my local area. I never would've thought it possible without this support. Thanks to you Fab you diamond"

—CAM DEMPSTER

Collaboration is not just about what you can do for someone else (or what someone can do for you), but it is also about being able to support and celebrate other people's victories. 80% of *highly influential people* agree that they strongly believe in celebrating their peers' successes.[64]

A considerable difference I found when looking at the two groups, is how both groups of influencers admit to being open to learn and share knowledge with people they respect and admire, but *highly influential people* are actively collaborating and cross-promoting on a regular basis other people in the industry they admire.[65]

Collaboration is also conducive of accountability between members of a community.

Social influencers have admitted to struggling with not having some form of accountability set in place to keep them on track with work. Having somebody to hold you accountable is something *highly influential people* are very aware of and actively seek. Bouncing ideas off other community members also entails sharing individual problems with one another. Often, we're terrified of admitting our problems or mistakes, but the only way we can solve them is to share them and recruit others to help us - it is a big test of vulnerability and humbleness.

Collaboration is something that has always been prevalent among artists. If you are willing to see yourself as a freelancer's content creator, the same way artists and philosophers view themselves then you're on the right track as they were the first ones to see the value of accountability among peers.

There is a misconception about artists, and that is the one that sees them as the lone wolfs - but this could not be further from the truth and oftentimes have accountability buddies holding them responsible. For example, philosopher Jean-Paul Sartre and Simone de Beauvoir were one such duo. Philosopher Karl Marx was not only the good friend and colleague of Friedrich Engels but often relied on him for regular handouts to support him in times of hardship.

But as well as collaborating for work, many creators emphasised the importance of friends and partners, who often help with the more practical and mundane parts of life. For example, Immanuel Kant would visit his best friend Joseph Green each day after his afternoon walk and would stay for a few hours to talk with him.

Interaction and accountability are important aspects of growing your influence within your community, and the key aspects of being a great leader. In fact, in a study called *Leading Collaboration in Online Communities,*[66] it's theorised that once members of an online community interact, the leadership roles blur thanks to the highly active nature of the community itself. You can, therefore, start training your leadership skills by just being an active member of a community.

Creating a community with a shared cause with Rupy Aujla

Dr Rupy Aujla, author, medical doctor, writer and podcaster has been making waves since setting up his blog, *Doctor's Kitchen.* In his latest venture, he is looking to bring Culinary Medicine to the UK. Culinary medicine is an evidence-based field in medicine combining the art of food and cooking with the science of medicine.

Culinary Medicine is aimed at helping people reach good personal medical decisions about accessing and eating high-quality meals that help prevent and treat disease and restore well-being.[67]

I asked Rupy to tell me more, and he gladly shared his vision (whilst making breakfast in his kitchen, very much on brand).

Here's Rupy's take on building a community and the power of collaborations:

Culinary Medicine is not new, it has been in the literature now for 12 years or so. Tulane Medical School, which is based in New Orleans, Louisiana started their Culinary Medicine program 6 years ago.

I reached out to them a year and a half ago, and I said: "Look, nobody is doing anything like this in the UK and it's something that really needs to happen. We need to educate our doctors in the foundation of nutrition, as well as how to cook."

I got sent their licensed media course, updated it for the UK audience, and started building the community. It's been a very slow progression, then I reached out to appropriate accreditation bodies for qualified GPs and basically tried to make it part of the curriculum.

What I am trying to achieve is basically a cultural change around food and medicine. I want people to be able to have an honest conversation about food and lifestyle with your GP, health professional or anyone within the community as it's very important.

I have managed to bring people together using social media, people within the food industry just to start the conversation and see who will be willing to help me. Initially, I had over 150 people reaching out. I narrowed it down to nine core people who will turn up to the meetings, engage and join the Slack group.

Everyone is volunteering their time at the moment, but I imagine in the future if we can get sponsorship we can grow this as a professional organisation that is not for profit.

I am really lucky that people show up and people are willing to donate their time I think that is partly because the vision is so grand.

We are aspirational, and everyone knows this needs to happen. I am also a hype man: I can hype things up, I am a good salesperson. I believe in something I can convey that enthusiasm and positivity to a group of people whether it's YouTube or a talk.

> I am very aware I have been able to harness that power and inspire this whole group of people to do that, and other people around me. This does not just come from being a good salesperson or having a genuine belief, but also being able to convey that in a structured way.

I am lucky to have these people (GPs and health professionals) who want to help me on my mission at the same time. We are really lucky to work in a collaborative industry, where people are willing to help each other, and certainly, the people I want to continue to liaise with are of a very collaborative nature.

This is so important, and that's why I am such a fan of making connections. Not just by being part of the community and benefitting from it, but also connecting people within the community.

Perhaps that's my personality, perhaps I believe in karma, as it's because these things come around and genuinely love it when people make a connection, and benefit themselves from me making that connection, as this is only adding to the community - which is a good thing.

My podcast is also linking up a lot of people: I am lucky that over the last couple of years I managed to meet a lot of people via Instagram, social media and my network and invite them on. Getting them on the podcast by having open conversations about food and medicine has been brilliant. So many people have been resonating with the podcast, as it has been downloaded over 150,000 times (at the time of the interview) and it's been supporting the book, as well as everything else. I think it is a very good resource and tool - I have not done a lot of episodes to this date, because I am all about quality - I want to be able to explain why every episode is so important and what you can get out of them.

I believe the biggest impact I am going to have is with Culinary Medicine. My goal is to establish Culinary Medicine. in the UK so that when students go to medical school they have a Culinary Medicine program and that will be because of the work I am slogging away at right now.

I am not benefiting from this, it's purely a passion, and it's a non-profit organisation I have started. It's changing the way seniors and juniors at college will look at food in the future. We'll change the conversation with our patients around food because it's the most impactful change we can make.

Whatever's your doctor tells you to change you will do, and this is why I am so passionate about this. The research is there, the passion is there: we are just not doing what we are taught to do.

On letting go of the Imposter Syndrome

You know those analogies that really stick with you, and you wish you knew where they came from? This is a bit how I feel about the story I am about to tell. A lot of people may be reading the examples and case studies in this book, and they may get triggered by the little voice in their heads - let's call it Arthur.

Arthur may be starting to say things like "well, you are no Hazel Wallace, so how do you think you can even make an impact on anyone?"

Here's where this analogy works so well, because life is, well, just like a flight of stairs.

Yes, I can feel your eyes rolling because that metaphor has been used a thousand times before; however, everyone is standing on a step in this gigantic flight of stairs - and trust me, you are far from being at the bottom.

When you feel you are not inspiring millions, think about the hundreds of people that are just one step below you.

These people are looking up to you, because you are, objectively, where they want to be. Never underestimate the impact you may have on the people around you, and remember, it's not about where you are in this flight of stairs compared to others, but it's about how can you inspire the ones below you to get there.

As the online community continues to grow and thrive, this presents a complex situation, in that it tells us there is growing interest and demand for the message (Double 'Woo!') And yet, for those of you creating content and wanting to share your voice, it also means there is A LOT of content to compare to.

Seeing what others are doing, writing, saying and creating can be a wonderful source of inspiration for us to interpret into our own vibe and enhance our own healthy viewpoint, as well as feel like we're part of a movement, so comparison isn't all bad.

Unfortunately, however, being inspired is not always the first thing can comes up to mind and, more often than not, comparison makes us look at other influencers and feel isolated and separate from them and, in many cases, we can develop secret rivalries, pitting ourselves against one another and competing in the ranks of Insta followers and Facebook likes and shares, and that's before we've even got on to book sales.

Despite being quite experienced with the concept of comparison myself, I decided to turn to one of my dearest and old friends for help in that department.

I met Lucy almost five years ago at a meet-up in Camden: it was a close group of girls, meeting up to share their hopes and dreams about turning the world into a better place. There she was, the adorable, funny and kind Lucy - with her Northern accent and unicorn halo.

Little did I know she'd become the first (and only) comparison coach. What is a comparison coach, Dear Reader? I am glad you asked.

Sabotage Alert: Comparison and influence with Lucy Sheridan

I am the world's first and only Comparison Coach which means my work is entirely focused on helping people get and stay in their own lane. I am also a golden retriever obsessed history geek (but I'm not sure how relevant that is!)

> *"I have made exploring and curing comparison my specialism having been severely affected from a young age."*

As a five-year-old, I remember looking at my newly born brother wondering if I was as cute as he was. Then in my school years, I made spelling tests and swimming badges a source of comparison and the ranking continued through my adolescence and into adulthood where I continued to pit myself against other people in an imaginary game of 'who is winning?', looking to others for markers and validation that I was doing OK.

My comparison crescendo came in my late twenties after I attended a reunion. The day itself was fun, and the prosecco flowed with the conversation as we nostalgically swapped stories into the night. It felt like the elixir of nostalgia took hold as we recounted younger years and I was able to forget what was going on in my life as, for me, things were far from perfect or worthy of comment.

My boyfriend's (now husband) business had been hit hard by the recession, and as a consequence, I felt like I was watching a car crash in slow motion as the worst thing we feared would happen became our reality. We were losing our house from under us, and I was holding myself together by a thin thread despite smiling and laughing along with the party atmosphere of the reunion.

As I stood surrounded by people that seemed to have it all sorted in their lives, what I could not have anticipated at the time, was those real-life interactions and conversations, would translate to accept friend requests that would triple my social networks overnight. In my vulnerable state, this was like fuel to my fire. With more people on my friends list, my sources of comparison and consumption habits went into overdrive, and I scrolled into a hole so deep and dark I completely forgot who I was, where I was going and what I wanted in my own life. From there, the only place was down, and my own comparing habits took an obsessive turn.

I would see a 'Fitspo' picture on Instagram and stand for an hour in front of the mirror comparing every line and limb of my own body. I lasered in on three people whose social feeds I would regularly check to keep tabs on how they were progressing. I saved and stored information about people, sometimes taking screenshots of their feeds so I could remind myself what they were achieving. If my curiosity was really piqued, I would go out of my way to stimulate conversations with people just so I could get more dirt on a certain person or scenario I had read about online. My comparison complex made it my business to know other people's business, and yet, do absolutely nothing about it.

It was on a Saturday afternoon two years later that things changed. I remember I had scrolled back through three years of someone's Facebook photos and rolled my eyes at him posting he was visiting the Maldives (again!) when my phone overheated in my hand and the screen went dead. Comparison had literally become too hot for me to handle. How did I end up here? Feeling so inferior, so lost, so inadequate and so unsure of myself, compared to my peers? To everyone, if I'm honest.

And then it dawned on me if I could think and feel myself into this, could I think and feel myself out of it and reconnect with myself? I had to at least try.

Initially, this personal assignment took me to easy-to-access resources like TED Talks and the bookshop's self-help aisle, then I signed up for online classes and subscribed to psychology blogs to gain a deeper view. The more I understood about myself and what motivated me – what I feared and where I wanted to be without anyone's influence – the more I noticed comparison loosen its grip. Despite my high pressured full-time job, which left very little time for personal interests, I found myself on 6am trains travelling across the country at weekends to attend life-coaching seminars, culminating in getting a loan to invest in my own coaching training.

Fast forward to today, and I have helped thousands of people dissolve their comparison complex and reclaim ownership of their thoughts and decisions. Whether I have coached them on Skype or in person, my clients have included pop stars and pub owners, Harry Potter actors and hair stylists, school children right through to retirees.

Do you think influencers and online figures are more prone to be a victim of the comparison trap?

It is still common to compare ourselves to people and progress offline and yet, yes, if a proportion of your time is spent on social media channels, your business runs on the internet, and you are required to be active online then there are so many more opportunities to fall in comparison traps.

There are a few reasons, or example:

1. On a very practical level, there are more people and accounts to notice

2. Social media is a huge part of the day job so although management of online time is possible, turning off completely, delegating or detoxing is often impossible.

3. By the very nature of the term 'influencer', it is suggesting that in this role you must have a look or a vibe or an opinion of your own so you can shape other people's views and worlds.

Each of us is having to march to the beat of that drum and yet face the challenge of doing it in our own way. There are examples of other people excelling and doing well everywhere, so it is all too easy to compare and feel like you are falling behind.

What is the first step to recognising they are stuck in a comparison rut?

Notice it and acknowledge it. If you can recognise you have been triggered it means you can do something about it. Also, don't judge it. Comparison may be an ugly side of human nature but it is still part of human nature so to try and pretend it isn't happening or judging yourself harshly is not helpful and actually stops you getting through it.

The next step is to look at how you can reconnect yourself with your own goals and dreams as this cuts off the oxygen to comparison.

How do you think comparison can spark among a community setting and your peers?

If one person or a clique of people are seen to be better or more successful than others, then this can cause comparison especially if everyone was once perceived to be on a certain level. For example, if you started blogging around the same time as someone else and suddenly their social media following takes off or they start getting brand deals out of nowhere this will prompt comparison as you gauge yourself against what they are achieving.

Do you think Instagram can be conducive to some of these negative feelings and behaviours?

Yes and yet if it were not Instagram, it would be another channel. We are curious creatures that like to people watch and keep tabs on each other, and yet this can often shine our light on our own shortcomings.

The negative feelings include:

- Envy -where we can't be supportive or positive about our comparison trigger because we resent them so much and we think they are undeserving

- Low self-confidence - when we compare and feel like. Failure because we have not progressed like the other person

- Confusion - as we obsess over other people's accomplishments we lose track of our own plans and doubt our own abilities and potential

What is the one thing you can do to be more aware of your feelings?

Remember that if someone has achieved what you want, it means it is possible, and your job is to trust the timing of your life and let your own path unfold. You are unique, and it will happen in its own way for you.

Habit Five: Cultivate a Learner Mindset

The Learner Mindset

"You don't learn to walk by following rules. You learn by doing, and by falling over."

—RICHARD BRANSON

Whilst doing my research, I stumbled upon a particularly fascinating book: The Talent Code,[68] by bestselling author Daniel Coyle. The book uses cutting-edge neurological research to "crack the talent code" and provide the reader with the three key factors behind the development of every talent: deep practice, ignition (or motivation) and master coaching.

Now, I must add that the book goes heavily into the link between neural pathways and our learning process. Coyle states that talent is directly linked to myelin growth, which is the insulation that wraps around our neural circuits. To stimulate myelin growth, you have to practice at the very edge of your current abilities, to wilfully make mistakes and correct them.

Still with me? Cool, now, here's the next step.

Practise is not enough: talent is formed when deep practice is encouraged through long-term motivation and enforced through master coaching, or what I'll call, for the sake of the book, mentoring.

Why am I breaking down the code for talent? Because talent comes from practice, and practice allows us to learn. Among all the habits I highlighted and studied, the power of learning is one of the ones that both highly influential people and social influencers agree on. Marisa, from *Miss Marzipan,* shared with me why learning is so important for her:

"I try to work on the things I love and need. Learning programs and so on has always been a means to an end to me. I have an idea about what I want to create and learning the process of making that vision a reality is what keeps me motivated to try new things. When it comes to programs and technology, the only way I can learn is by doing. I am not interested in the mechanics of things generally, so technology in and of itself bores me. But if I imagine that a computer and program are no different to a sheet of paper and a pen (i.e., tools to create), then I can deal with it."

From reading this, it seems like Coyle was onto something. In order to learn you need to make mistakes, you need to be motivated, and you need to get guidance.

I talked about failing and making mistakes before, but it's something I do not think can be stressed enough: if you want to practice anything efficiently, don't shy away from your mistakes, but focus on adjusting them until you improve. Especially, I'd like to add, when it comes to things that do not come naturally to you.

For example, I am the artist. I am the maverick, the hyperactive creator who learns from doing. University settings have been incredibly hard for me, especially when I was learning by repeating some long lucubrations mechanically from literary critics (how my teacher thought that was going to benefit me later in my life is beyond me).

As I came to the UK for my year abroad, I did open myself up to a whole new way of learning: enter the essays.

Needless to say - I loved essays. They are basically mini-books which allowed me to get obsessed about a specific topic (see a pattern here?).

I learnt how to write essays without having had any sort of teaching (the perks of going abroad and having to get accustomed to a new education system), but that was the first instance of me learning about my limits and the challenges in my way of assimilating information.

As I mentioned in a previous example, my most challenging learning environment was during my PT course - there I faced another incredibly hard hurdle. The theory. The science. The body. I simply could not get it in my head. I would look at the diagrams and illustrations and eventually figure out how my heart works. You probably would have not wanted me to perform you a CPR back then.

Nevertheless, I was an absolute star at coaching my fellow colleagues, figuring out how the machine worked, and creating programs. Anatomy and physiology kept me awake most nights. I had to write things five times in five different ways, I had to wait until the proverbial penny dropped from the top of a six-stories building before I could even understand some of what I was reading.

Did I pass my exams? Yep, all at the first attempt (once again, geek).

Was it an easy feat? Absolutely not.

You'll have to get out of your comfort zone to keep your brain active and learning, and challenging itself. Practise is such an important aspect of learning.

As I mentioned before, Nobel laureate Herbert Simon[69] argues that it takes around 10,000 hours (or roughly ten years) to become an expert in a subject. After ten years of practice, around 50,000 chunks of knowledge become internalised in the brain, meaning that we can process them automatically. This knowledge becomes readily accessible to the brain without us having to really think about it - just like an expert football or tennis player would do.

I am not advocating it being a done science, neither would I say the outcome of the study is going to be objectively true for everyone. However, I do feel like it took me 10,000 hours to figure out what the heck the aorta is doing on a daily basis.

As I keep saying "repetition is the mother of skills". By practising beyond the limits of our current abilities, we encourage what Coyle called deep practice.

Why does practice need to be deep? Coyles argues that even the skill required to perform the simplest action demands thousands of nerves firing in perfect synchrony. [70]The more we repeat a task, the more precise and quick the action will become, because the myelin layer surrounding the relevant circuit thickens.

I have been blessed in my family with both my Grandad and my Brother being self-taught musicians.

My Grandad could play five different instruments. I asked him to teach me more than once, but his answer would always be the same "I have nothing to teach you that you cannot learn yourself". I'd sit next to him whilst he was playing, trying to replicate some of my favourite songs. When you are fully immersed in the environment, culture or world you want to learn from, learning becomes almost second nature.

By creating a structure that allows you to create a feasible, structured way of learning (for more information about breaking big tasks into chunks, head back to habit one, when talking about breaking goals into smaller tasks). Make sure you are looking at the task as a whole, then breaking it down into very small units. This will also allow you to slow down your pace, and therefore learn more effectively.

Another important aspect of learning is the motivation that propels you to go forward. That tiny voice that keeps telling you it's all worth it. This is also why I am not a massive fan of learning-overload.

Commit to a new skill, practice or course and let that be your sole focus until you feel you are at the level you wish to get to. Motivation gets diluted, tiredness and discouragement kick in, and it's harder to follow through - *highly influential people* seem to agree with me, 70% of them are starting to be "sort of obsessed with a specific topic right now, and that obsession helps me succeed".

Become obsessed with learning first, and then become obsessed with what you are learning.

Who are your mentors?

Some people may argue mentors are around us at all times - which is something I can get behind - but I do believe in finding specific mentors is an essential part of anyone's journey. Whether it is a teacher, a coach, or simply someone who is willing to help you develop your vision and grow your influence, mentors are the ones that will support you with your learning process.

Almost no one develops their talents by themselves - teachers and coaches can support us with the motivation required to practise our skills. The beauty of the world today is that teachers come in different shapes and forms.

They can be someone we follow, learn from and read about passively, without necessarily having met them. It can be someone who is willing to show you how to grow your skills or simply a personal tutor. It can even be someone that you are related to.

So, how do you go about finding a mentor?

The best thing is, nine times out of ten, just ask somebody out for a coffee.

If you are looking for a coach or a mentoring figure that can provide you with accountability, I recommend going to friends and peers in the community and ask for recommendations. This is how I started mentoring bloggers and influencers again. People kept coming to me asking me for someone who could mentor them, and at some point, I had to throw in the towel and accept that the Universe wanted me to be that figure for them.

Another way to find mentors is to look at your current teachers and tutors and ask them for some personal feedback or advice.

I still remember my literature teacher fondly. She was very strict, and most of the class was not necessarily a big fan of hers. However, dork alert, I really loved literature and her way of teaching it to us. One day I came to her telling her I wanted to be a writer. One thing leads to another, and I ended up handing her a manuscript for one of my short stories, probably not expecting a lot out of it.

A few days later she came back with the pieces of paper, scribbled all over and highlighted in almost every direction. This was the beginning of a long correspondence. It actually makes me quite emotional to think back at this because she truly believed in me. She believed in my passion, and my enthusiasm, and prompted me to write more, branch out, and not give up.

This is what a mentor should be. They should be there to celebrate your successes and push you to be inherently better.

No matter where you find them, let your mentors be the ones that can push you to higher heights. Someone who still does that, despite no longer being with us, is my Grandad - as you know, I consider him a big influencer of mine.

Since I was very young, he was the one who transmitted his passions to my brother and me. My Grandad was everything I aspired to be: talented, creative, active, charming. What I was not necessarily as fond of was how he would constantly take my gullibility to higher heights, by testing how many of his bizarre stories and fantasies I would believe. Unsurprisingly, most of them.

He did teach me a lot of things though, without even trying.

What I loved about my grandad was his innate ability to make everyone feel special - whether it was by stealing a smile off them, or complimenting them.

He was the flirtiest man I have ever met, and his charm definitely helped him with that. I remember him once telling a young woman that he was 90 years old. "No Grandad!. You're only 75!" I informed him. "Well, you won't get compliments off ladies if you say you are 75, will you?" he winked.

It's probably because of him that I learnt not to take myself too seriously - that, at the end of the day, people will love you and relate to you because of who you are. I also embraced the "no filters" attitude and the hyper-ness, which sometimes does frustrate people.

My Grandad believed that being a better person for others would make you happier. (He also believed that water made you rusty - as I said, nobody is perfect).

Another thing I learnt from him was to be passionate. My Grandad was a keen tennis player, a soccer coach, a multi-instrumentalist and a painter. I remember us dancing around the vinyl player like maniacs listening to Frank Sinatra and Liza Minelli.

"Giorgio, you are going to hurt yourself!" my Grandma would shout covering her face, while we engaged in little twist moves.

As someone who was growing up feeling the urge to impress and be loved, I looked up to Gramps and wanted him to be proud of me. The excitement of showing him I learnt to play "Stand by Me" all by myself was immense. He was my hero, after all.

"Babette, Babette!" he would call me from the other room while looking at old photos.

He would tell me stories about the old times - he said that it was important to pass along the knowledge, to keep stories alive. He may not have been a writer, but he was onto something.

Some days I miss him, very much. The way he would show me how to light up his pipe. His frugality - which would irrevocably upset my Mum. The way he was loved by everyone, and how he could get out the right joke at the right time - clockwork almost.

My Grandad taught me to be creative. Question things. Pass along knowledge. Tell stories that need to be told. Be passionate. Love music. Be kind and make people feel good.

Every time I go down to see hello to him I sit on his tombstone and I tell him about all the crazy things that have changed. In those moments I can see myself and my Nonno picking up berries, up in the mountains.

"See this berry" he'd say, holding the tiniest strawberry.

"Yes", I'd reply.

"It was there, in those bushes, hidden. Always look out for the small things, and hold onto them."

Learning and self-development

"Why are you learning what you are learning?" I asked Niki from *Rebel Recipes* about why she decided to study as a health coach. Her response was rather telling:

> *"It's something I thought about for a long time before deciding to study. Two main reasons: Enhance my nutritional knowledge more formally, i.e. get a qualification. The holistic approach to health is very important to me. I wanted to develop my coaching skills. For myself and others." Whatever it is that you want to improve, you'll only get there if you change yourself first. If you remember in the first part of this book we talked about habits - the best way to achieve lasting personal change is to develop better habits.*

Habits shape us. Not only how we act, but who we are, is, to a large extent, defined by our habits. By making learning a new habit, you can include it in your daily routine without making it yet another task in your to-do list.

Learning should be as much your drive to grow as a person, as it should be your interest in widening your horizons. Learning is, after all, a very fine form of self-development.

When Stephen Covey, author of *7 Habits of Highly Effective People*, embarked on his quest to truly understand the nature of success, he began by immersing himself in some 200 years' worth of literature on the topic, starting from 1776.[71]

Based on his study he concluded that, generally speaking, there are two ways to strive for improvements to your life: the first method is to work on the skills necessary for the behaviour you desire. This is what we see more often when wanting to develop any kind of personal skills - for example, if you are looking to deliver speeches in public, you'll work on your communication skills. This is what he calls the personality ethic: a method particularly popular since the 1920s but very often considered a shortcut. A lot of people use this method instead of working on their character and therefore miss an incredibly valuable piece of the puzzle when it comes to the learning experience.

In all truthfulness, the second method, which focuses on your core habits and belief systems, is what should be addressed first. Covey argues that working on your beliefs should be paramount. Once you are able to recognise and analyse the beliefs that form your view of the world, you'll be able to understand which skills you want to develop, and for which purpose. This aspect, called the character ethic, encourages people to get clear on which values they want to prioritise in their life, such as courage, integrity and the golden rule.

This approach is the one that has been identified before the 1920s, for example, in the writings of Benjamin Franklin;[72] use what you learn as a way to learn more about yourself, and subsequently learn new skills enrich your knowledge base and overall feed into your expertise and grow credibility.

As Hannah and Emily from *Twice the Health* shared with me when discussing the dynamic or working together as a pair, they admitted: "We are both very aware of our strengths and weaknesses, and luckily a lot of our weaknesses can be strengthened by the other's skills. It's not always easy, but we are certainly getting better at listening to each other and recognising who knows best. We can both be a little stubborn, but I guess that's something to work on right? "

Let me add this though: all the PhDs in the world will not stand the test of time if you do not allow yourself to learn exactly who you are, what your core values are, and how you want to enrich the world through them.

I recommend everyone to revise their core values at least every six months. Values can be family, love, commitment, freedom, success, expansion and so on. Learning can often be mistaken as the need to learn something new about the world when most often the best learning we can do is the one about ourselves.

The best learning happens outside the classroom

"Tell me, and I forget. Teach me, and I remember. Involve me, and I learn."

—BENJAMIN FRANKLIN

As I've mentioned a few time before, I am an avid reader. As I was reading Tim Ferris' *Tools of Titans,* Chris Sacca mentioned his "Sweet and Sour Summers". This reminded me of my own version of summer internships - and what these have taught me about life.

As I mentioned at the beginning of this section, learning is not always something that will be delivered in a classroom. But let me start from the very beginning.

In Italy, especially in my region, working in and around the countryside is a thing. Think about the rural farm experience: picking fruit, or helping in vineyards, or whatever may be needed. I was lucky to know a few farmers and to be needing a new laptop for my writing endeavours. I knew I could have asked for one for my birthday, but I wanted to feel what it'd be like to work for it - something that'd become a thread throughout my University years.

Despite my parents not finding it necessary for me to spend one and a half months working out in the sun after finishing my exams, I shrugged shoulders and said: "well, I'll be able to get my own laptop, so how bad can this be".

I picked pears for two summers. Six days a week, starting at 8am and finishing at around 6pm each day. Sometimes we would even do Sunday shifts if required. We were paid minimum wage and only allowed a small break. If it does not sound fun, it's because it wasn't. It was tedious, never-ending and quite honestly mind-numbing (I did get to drive the truck a few times though). There was a time during the day where the sun was directly above you, and the bushes would not provide any shadow - literally what the term "nowhere to hide" was invented for. That usually would last for the two hours around lunchtime - and if that does not teach you the value of resilience, I do not know what does.

Everyone had to do specific chores depending on the day; carry wooden boxes, drag small carts with more wooden boxes, or jump on and off small trucks in the mud (once again, as dangerous as it was fun). Still, I survived every push, every pull and every sweaty tear.

Picking up pears is especially tricky as you have different categories and different ways of storing each pear. A bush can have up to 25 pears, each of them needing to be checked and classified in one of the different categories. I needed to be a good observer and extremely patient.

Some days, we'd spend hours in silence, and others were spent listening to Iron Maiden through very tiny speakers.

There were not many distractions, so in a way, it was quite a Zen-like experience. At the time I had my end goal in mind, and little else really. Patience, focus and efficiency became three important factors when it came to doing a great job.

I showed up every morning with a great attitude. I did this because no matter what job you are in, you have to show up 100%. I did it equally when giving tuitions, serving chicken, making lattes (very poorly, most likely one of the most scarring experiences of my life).

If there is one thing that those Summers taught me it was that some days you are going to feel like a boss, some days you'll have to carry big boxes in the rain. And that's okay. The truth is, a lot of the skills you've learnt will be transferred to your future self.

"Lots of my skills have been transferable such as project management, structure, managing multiple projects etc.", Niki Webster pointed out.

If that's something I know I'll be wanting my own children to experience, is being able to get their hands dirty. Do the simple jobs, just never forget to work towards whichever goal may be at the finish line. Because once you learn how to be genuinely excited about waking up at 6am to pick up fruits without really complaining, you'll be much more excited about a lot of things that life will present you with.

Become obsessed with learning

When it came to the research I carried out, I noticed that the topic of learning and investing in yourself was the topic with the most validations. This was no surprise as *highly influential people* do value investing in themselves: "I invest money and time learning from people I admire" is something pretty much everyone unanimously agreed on.

Niki Webster shared with me why she decided to keep on her studies from her health coach course to her recent raw chef course:

"I thought about for a long time before deciding to enrol my health coaching program. Two main reasons were to enhance my nutritional knowledge more formally; i.e. get a qualification. The holistic approach to health is critical to me. I wanted to develop my coaching skills. For myself and others."

Ways you can invest in yourself and your learning:

- Attend a seminar/workshop
- Join a course / start a degree
- Join a book club
- Listen to audiobooks
- Listen to podcasts

- Have a list of monthly books you want to read

- Join a mastermind

- Curate an RSS feed with your favourite publications

As I mentioned a few times before already, learning comes in many forms and should be approached as a way to keep up with what is happening around you.

Whether you decide to completely change your current focus or to add more value to something you are already invested in (such as a degree, an additional course or a specialisation.

Becoming obsessed with learning is something all influencers have in common.

This comes back to the fact that if you want to tell a story, create something for your community and audience that can also revive the trust and credibility, you have to know what you are talking about.

I wish I could tell you there will be a time when you can stop learning - but to live we have to evolve and to evolve, we have to keep on learning. It's easy to use 'busy' as our over encompassing excuse for not being able to spend some time learning something new, however, just like I presented when discussing the concept of habits, it's easy to fall out of the practice itself, and this is when learning is no more an enjoyable activity but a chore.

I say this because the practice of reading news and trends for me is a very effective, simple and stimulating way of reviving the learning spark and the passion for the industry I am in.

Influencers are trend-setters, and as such people are looking up to them to hear, see and get inspired by the latest trends, products or even strategies they have tried and tested. This is why, as an influencer, learning can be something you do in so many different ways at any given time.

Remember, the idea is that by influencing people you are also inspiring them to take up new habits and grow as individuals. Learning is such a key aspect, yet something that so overlooked due to the way influencers are perceived nowadays.

You can take the most mind-blowing pictures of yourself in front of a tropical paradise, but if you do not strive to improve, learn and challenge your beliefs you are, ultimately not bringing anything new to the space itself.

As I mentioned multiple times throughout this book, your aim should be to make a positive impact. Dream big and bold, and work hard for it.

Why you have your best ideas in the shower

You know the old saying "I always happen to have my best ideas in the shower". Well, guess what, there is a reason for that.

How can we have a clear idea of what creativity does to our brain?

Researchers Allen Braun and Siyuan Liu had a genius idea: track the brain activity of rappers doing freestyle.[73]

Why freestyle?

It's easy to track, it's a very creative process, and it tends to happen very quickly (if you do not believe me, watch a few epic rap battles on YouTube).

When we are creative, some of the brain areas we use for everyday decisions are entirely deactivated, while others we don't use will light up:

> *"Artists showed lower activity in part of their frontal lobes called the dorsolateral prefrontal cortex during improvisation, and increased activity in another area called the medial prefrontal cortex. The areas that were found to be 'deactivated' are associated with regulating other brain functions."*

For the first time, researchers have been able to analyse an activity that would be called 'creative' and actually measure its impact. When it comes to the "medial prefrontal cortex" area, this is the area which is responsible for learning association, context, events and emotional responses.

Once again, to let Braun explain to us what this means:

> *"We think what we see is a relaxation of 'executive functions' to allow more natural de-focused attention and uncensored processes to occur that might be the hallmark of creativity."*

I know what you must be thinking, Dear Reader: "Fab, this still is not really telling me why I have great ideas in the shower".

Let's be honest, showers are NOT that creative. However, they help us with our dear old friend (and scientific brain chemical) dopamine. Yes, an essential ingredient for us to be creative is dopamine. The more dopamine that is released, the more creative we are. Or, at least, that's what Braun says: "People vary concerning their creative drive according to the activity of the dopamine pathways of the limbic system."[74]

Dopamine levels rise when we are energised, inspired or relaxed. Let's be honest, warm showers and hot baths can be extremely relaxing. Once again though, if that's the case, we'd be creative even when planking or doing squats.

Another important part of learning and the creative process is novelty. Learning something new instigates novelty: it stimulates our brain, especially when learning something new, as it builds connections between neurons, replacing some of those we lose over time.

Welcome to the world of "neuroplasticity" - a world which I dipped into for the purpose of this book, and my very own brain struggled to keep up with it. This is basically where neuron stimuli, dopamine, and neurotransmitters come together. Neuroplasticity is sparked from a combination of all the elements that support the creative process (such as dopamine, novelty, learning), and helps our brain evolving, changing and challenging itself. However, there is one last piece of this puzzle: distraction.

Now, I can get distracted incredibly easily: a cute baby (or a baby sloth crawling in the grass) will always do the trick. However, not all distractions are equal. This time is the time Shelley H. Carson, author of *Your Creative Brain*, calls incubation period. She adds: "a distraction may provide the break you need to disengage from a fixation on the ineffective solution."[75]

Especially when thinking about something that is deeply buried in our subconscious mind, as soon as you let your mind wander, it can surface and plant those ideas into your conscious mind. For that, showers are indeed one way to learn and be creative, and I also recommend going for a walk.

It's no surprise that loads of leaders, such as Arianna Huffington, have been employing very similar tools such as walking meetings for years now. I tend to do the same; walking phone calls, walking podcast strolls, walking to solve problems.

As per usual, I was curious to see the reason why walking is such a creativity tool. A study developed in Stanford University demonstrated that walking boosts creativity thanks to the clear mind-body connection. It opens up the free flow of ideas, the effect is not simply due to the perceptual stimulation of moving through an environment, but rather it is due to walking.[76]

The takeaway from this is very simple: learning should not be confined to a classroom environment. Development and growth should be encouraged in whichever environment works for you.

Being able to create prime learning environments for yourself can both implement and increase the joy of learning in itself, and inspire creativity through learning. Being able to turn the learning experience into an investment is what can make a difference in the way you spread your very own message.

How books can spark your creative Mojo with Shelf Help

Sometimes you meet the best people almost by accident. This is pretty much how it felt like with Toni Jones. After quite a long Insta-stalking activity, Toni and I managed to meet, in real life (like the cool kids do), in the beautiful Ibiza.

At the time we met, Toni just started her venture, Shelf Help, and I was incredibly excited to see her taking the idea of Shelf Help and develop it into what it is today.

But what is Shelf Help?

Shelf Help is a book club dedicated to self-help books. Its mission is to make self-help more accessible and to connect as many people as possible with life-changing books.

"Self-help books and support groups had a huge impact on me at a pretty tough time in my life, and the idea behind Shelf Help is to combine the two to create safe spaces (online and offline) for people to come together and support each other at the same time as developing themselves. Because I believe the reason we are ALL here is to learn and grow into the best version of ourselves."

Why do you think self-help books are such an important asset when it comes to learning and self-development?

Self-help is such a broad genre that it covers every aspect of our lives - emotional, physical, mental and spiritual - and there is absolutely something for everyone. Books have always been a beautiful way to pass on information and ideas because we can really get lost in them, and I believe the right book(s) can really change our lives as they challenge the way we think and behave and then ultimately live.

> *"Books, Kindle, audible, Instagram - all great learning tools. I love that books can be shared."*

How do you think learning new skills and engaging in different topics outside of our comfort zone can really help us?

The only way we EVER grow is by taking ourselves out of our comfort zones, and so it's something we should be doing all the time, whether that's through books or experiences or people. Lots of us are desperate to know why we're here and what our purpose is and the best way to find that out is by trying LOTS of things - and to keep doing that our whole lives.

How can different skills learn through reading enriching us when it comes to the way we approach life and work?

The more we read, the more we learn, the more we question, listen and grow. Challenging our limiting behaviours and learning to master our thoughts and emotions through reading helps us dream bigger, be more and live better. And isn't that what it's all about?

Habit Six:
Be More Vulnerable

Be selfless by being selfish

A few years back I remember talking to my editor (and at the time overall right hand gal), Laura. We were discussing my tasks and commitments throughout the week ahead.

"All right, so, 45 hours on the HBC, then the blog, hum the newsletter and the PT stuff..." As the note-taker of the business, Laura kept scribbling and doing the maths. She looked up and asked, "Would you say another 15 for your PT clients?"

"Yeah I guess that is accurate", I replied, trying to keep up with my very own mental arithmetic skills.

"So that is 60 hours in total" she finally announced.

I raised my eyebrows, whilst internally my jaw dropped. Ah. Well, that was news to me.

Straight after that, my brain starts infiltrating other questions: "Did you count the time you spend on Instagram? What about those cheeky emails you send between the station and work?"

I felt physically sick. After all, didn't they tell me that if I do what you love then I'd never work one day in my life yet here I was working, at least, 60 hours per week?

The external and internal pressures can often feel much more intense than what we let others see.

Being self-employed (or double-employed) puts a lot of pressure on ones shoulders and overworking is not something that is really openly discussed. In fact, sometimes it can be romanticised.

I have been there. I was the always-busy business coach of financial freedom and a roaring advocate that passive income rocked, however, most of the time the amount of work that needed to go into achieving any of the above was clearly understated..

The moment of acceptance and realisation that I couldn't keep going at that pace made me feel physically sick.

However, that's when I realised that in order to grow, make a bigger impact (not to mention have the time to implement all the other habits I had been practicing) that I had to be "selfish" In fact, it was essential. There are a few straight forward ways to do so and being willing to ask for help is the biggest one. A few more ways include delegation and automation.

Delegate and bring people into your vision

The main obstacle when it comes to implementing delegation taking a leap of faith. This is true for our wallets and our control-freak minds alike. Type A people (like Yours Truly) know that delegating is important. But how quickly can we make up for that investment? And how can we be sure people will do as good a job as we would?

Delegating is both a mental and financial investment. As simple as that. Sometimes I made massive poops and hired people who would not fit - and found it 500 times harder to delegate again. However, I stopped seeing it as a loss, and I turned it into a gain - as I learnt more about business and how to liaise with employees, and just like in relationships, it teaches you what you are looking for in someone.

Let's be honest, we are being incredibly picky about our partners, so why would we not be the same about the people we have to see day in and day out?

For the purpose of this habit, I read a lot of research about hiring people. Everyone you want to bring into your vision has to be vetted effectively; from assistants to co-founders.

A lot of influencers start with a VA (Virtual Assistant).

The virtual assistant will basically organise your life and tackle all the tasks that are time consuming, mind-numbing (for a lack of a better word) and tedious. VAs and business partners are the roles you see cropping out a lot for influencers. VAs help you making your life easier, business partners support you when launching a side-project.

In a world where Instagram has taken over from a resume, I have to ask, are skills still the most relevant thing to look for in someone wanting to join your vision? Personally, there are other things I like to consider such as the individual's personality. I like to get very clear idea of the characteristics of the people I want to include the HBC vision. I always thought it was not as important as skills and numbers, however, it turns out that it is what makes or breaks the way you grow your influence.

Let's put it this way; just because you may not be a business yet it does not mean you should not value the hiring process. Hiring is often treated as a last-minute necessity and this approach brings in poor results. To make sure that your vision has the talent it needs to succeed, you should instead make hiring a top priority.

If you're someone who is considering taking over the world with your business on your own then you need to factor in being incredibly exhausted and ineffective most of the time. As Niki from *Rebel Recipe* points out when discussing the life of a freelancer: "the hardest part is not being part of a team and having people to bounce ideas off. I try to network as much as possible and have some amazing friends but I still miss being in a team."

There are many ways to find, vet and approve people, but I found a tool that works for me (and friends who have gone through the process) that there are a few key aspects to bear in mind - and just like magic, we're going through our past habits again!

Just like we mentioned in Habit One, you need to be clear on your vision, mission and messaging. Your tone, the way you want to communicate your message are something you need to be able to present to a stranger in the street in less than a minute. If you still cannot do that, you may want to wait before hiring someone.

I know that for both of my companies I am looking for fun, tongue-in-cheek, informative messages and communication. It's memorable, and should steal everyone a smile. People who can bring that to the mix are the winners for me.

This means - wait for it - that ensuring a cultural fit might mean saying no to people with serious talent. Just remember: a prospective hire might be incredible at their job, but not share your company's values and, in the end, your brand and your mission is more important than that.

Another important aspect comes from Habit Four and it's about harnessing your community. It's best to get referrals from your networks, both your community and private network. That's not just me saying it. Seventy-seven percent of the CEOs interviewed in *Who*,[77] a very interesting book about hiring and company culture, said that using their own network was hands down the best way to make successful hires for their company.

One of the key points when it comes to finding the right people, is to *always* be searching for people that seem to fit the bill, not just seeking them out when you know you need them. This saves you having a poll of people you are just half-way happy with at the time.

Let's say you find the right people.

Then what?

There are plenty of techniques and ways to vet your potential candidates, however, one of the things that is heavily overlooked is the importance of putting people in a position of having to complete a task.

Even better if you give them little instruction on the methods, and let them naturally show you how they'd tackle a specific situation.

Overall, you want to make sure you can work alongside someone, and being able to see them in action is the most important step of them all.

Boundaries. Boundaries. More boundaries.

I always worked hard to set boundaries for the HBC, however, it's not just about setting working hours or putting on your out-of-office because as highly connected humans we often want to answer emails in a heartbeat or answer a call from a good friend. In a world where we scroll Instagram 10 times per hour, boundaries are blurred and we don't even know it.

Especially when the dreaded feeling of failure kicks in and we begin to tell ourselves that if we work more then we'll achieve more and we begin to run around in circles. Furthermore, despite everything looking glossy in the magical world of social media, the bigger your influence gets, the more pressure you naturally put on yourself.

It is the basic concept of responsibility, as well as honour. However, kicking back may open more doors than expected. Truth is, it's never easy.

The universe challenges you in mysterious ways. For example, I remember once getting the phone call;

"You know that project you wanted so badly? Guess what? They accepted your proposal! You do not mind adding that to your plate, do you? And you'll have to handle it alone because your VA is getting married in the Galapagos next week!"

Huh?

When life throws you a curve ball (or two), you got to breathe deeply and move on. The main action you can take is setting better and stronger boundaries - here's a few ideas on how to do so:

- Set an autoresponder with clear email times or turnaround time

- Add clear working hours to any agreement you send

- Do not check your email before/after a certain time

- Take notifications off your phone

- Delete social / email apps that you cannot stop checking

In the meanwhile, there's one more thing you can do when things start feeling too much.

Ask for someone to listen. Whether it is a mastermind group, a peer friend, your partner - you got to let it out. No, do not lash out like a banshee. Most of the time the solution is already there, but you are too deeply engrossed in your thoughts to notice it.

To go back to the "love what you do and you'll never work a day in your life", we all know that working on something you truly love is infectious, and it's often hard to say no to. However, always remember that friendships, relationships and wanderlust are equally important.

It's not about work life balance, as much as it is about work-life boundaries - to quote Niki when asking her about finding balance:

> "I'm always working towards balance. I tend to prioritise work over everything else. It's important for me to incorporate time to train. It gives my day structure so ideally: yoga in the morning and

cardio or weights later. However, I don't worry if I don't have time to do that and I'm kinder to myself now. Spending time with friends and being in the countryside is also really important to me."

On being a busy Mum and successful blogger with Marisa from Miss Marzipan

I was thinking about all the mamas out there, growing their influence, working on amazing projects and raising kids. As women, we tend to be much clearer about what self-care means to us, and yet we don't give ourselves the time to indulge in it. Marisa, otherwise known as *Miss Marzipan* is a professional art director, recipe creator, stylist, visual communicator and food photographer.

This lady's content is stunning, and her commitment to the community and her work is second to none. I asked her a few questions about balance, family life and work ethic.

About Marisa

Eating well has provided me with so much more than just fuel and nutrients. Discovering a passion for cooking, for food and for living well has been a true joy. My first tentative and somewhat shaky cooking experiences led me to become determined to know more, to eat better… and to eat more.

A catalyst in my wellness journey was TTC (or 'trying to conceive' as it's known in non-TTC circles!). The road to motherhood was a long and bumpy one for me. Somewhere in amongst landing my "dream job", TTC, miscarriage and trying to improve my health, I was diagnosed with hypothyroidism (a condition that is thankfully stable these days). The subject of food became of increasing interest and I decided to go organic whenever possible.

The journey of whole foods and home cooking discovery continued throughout my pregnancy with my son, during which a sudden intense aversion to meat led me to experiment with vegetarian cooking. And then, during my high risk pregnancy with my daughter, all matters health and wellbeing-related were of primary importance to me.

We can't choose all the things life hands us, but if we are fortunate we can choose what we consume. And I don't think there's a rational person out there who would argue that eating wholesome, home cooked food is detrimental to health.

Personally, I have found a way to eat that works for me on many levels; one that feels health-affirming, exciting and genuinely enjoyable. I want my children to love food; to love what it gives them in terms of enjoyment and nourishment, to love knowing about it, to love cooking it.

What helps you being organised, have a clear outline of priorities and main focus for each week?

I wish I could say I did. I use a planner, but I am not always consistent. When I do use it, I prioritise the must-do and usually have 3 on the list. Anything else that gets ticked off is a bonus.

How do you make sure you keep a balanced approach to work and life, especially being a mama?

I actually involve my kids and husband a lot in what I do. They cook with me, they throw recipe ideas at me, they even help me shoot (I have showed my kids the basic functions of a camera and my husband is a talented creator who I met at art school). I keep what I do a family affair and in this way I can make the most of being a WAHM (Work at Home Mum) while also keeping things fun for my kids.

How do you strive balance throughout your week?

At the moment the best I can do is meditation in the morning (a few minutes), prioritising cuddles with the kids and eating meals as a family. Work is a 7 day per week thing right now, so balance is clearly not on point.

How do you make sure you make enough time for yourself?

I have minimums. Mine are daily meditation and drinking water (lemon water) before I consume anything else.

Other than that, I am not particularly great with this at the moment. My husband is very accommodating and will take the children out to give me some space and time, but I usually work. That's my honest answer.

In what ways do you make time for yourself and reset?

I love spa days. I don't have them enough of course. And when I am going to the gym, I really enjoy that. Not doing it at the moment though. Meditation of at least a couple of minutes is my bare minimum. It's a truly off day if I can't even manage that!

When being vulnerable is a form of Self-Care

"Because true belonging only happens when we present our authentic, imperfect selves to the world, our sense of belonging can never be greater than our level of self-acceptance."

—BRENE BROWN

I do not remember much about the months that followed my Dad's passing. I was stuck in a spiral of coping mechanisms and denial.

"You know, I just cannot cry", I said to my flatmate, as we were sitting next to each other watching Netflix.

"Oh that's great, I mean you're over it" she replied.

"I really want to cry", I said, "I really, really do."

I was fresh from too many changes, and desperately trying to cry. I started watching old Buffy episodes (spoiler alert: I mean the ones in which she dies, or Angel dies), or I put on old music from my teenage emo days. I even got my dark MOJO back and began writing gloomy poetry again.

One night, sitting in bed, I stared outside my window and had a conversation with my Grandad. Maybe I was just talking to myself but either way, it helped. I was reflecting on how much I've changed, specifically thanks to the fact that I was working on my own vision and my own mission.

Oh, Dear Reader, you may say "it was for the better" or "it was for the worse" - however, growing your influence and having a business changes you and shapes you in ways that you don't expect - and self-help books definitely don't talk enough about.

Since I embarked on my journey I have become much more upfront even with people that I don't know. So you can find me at the hairdresser talking about my past relationships, sharing my biggest worries about life and everything in-between. I used to be the girl who would never talk about her problems with friends, let alone strangers. I did feel a bit bad for the lady who had to wash my hair and cut it while I was going through my life story in depth.

The second thing that I noticed is that I take more chances.

Clear example: a few years back, I cut my hair so short that now I can literally dry my pixie crop by shaking it off. It was impulsive, it was new, and I went along with it. I became more open to try things that may not have worked before. You can either follow your intuition and go with your gut, or follow a strategy that has been put in front of you.

Lastly, I realised that whilst on this journey it's become really hard for me to be easy on myself. A friend of mine once said that instead of declaring that she is "too hard on herself", she will now start saying that she is "quite easy on herself". It was such an important step when it came to the way I'd accept my mistakes, flaws and failures of sort.

I constantly remind myself of how far I have come, and that despite having had a few *divine storms* in my time, and have found myself having to leave everything and start over again, I opened myself to others and asked for help.

Sometimes we see someone from the outside, and we think that they will never crack, however, more and more *highly influential people* realised that, just like Brene Brown said: *"Courage starts with showing up and letting ourselves be seen."*

A couple of days after that chat with my friend, I decided that I was going to stop and have an honest talk with myself and it went like this;

"I love you and you are allowed to be vulnerable" I said to the person in the mirror. "You are allowed to fall down and come back up, you're allowed to ask for help, you are allowed to be grumpy, and you are allowed to scream and shout and cry." I stopped, then I added, "Remember that I love you and I am proud of you".

That night, Dear Reader, was the night I cried.

A note on beliefs
and our self-talk

As I was rummaging around old writings of mine, I found a post I wrote with my unicorn onesie on (used to be my official this woman means business uniform). The post was about my Ideal Day and is a great exercise that usually helps you attract more good energy and positive outcomes into your life.

Well, I ended up going to bed pretty distressed, with a mountain of scrapped paper.

Instead of following my intuition, the post ended up being about what I was "supposed" to do or where I was "supposed" to live. I was thinking about economising and practicality.

Ah, that's it.

How can you economise on your ideal life? I am all about minimalism and simplicity, but I had to stop a second and ask myself: am I doing this from a place of fear?

For a long while, I convinced myself that I was living in the now in order to be more aware rather than working on a Virgos idea of a 4 years plan. It turns out that some of us use the term "living in the now".

I decided to let go of some of my religious beliefs, and started exploring other religions such as Buddhism where I stumbled about the concept of impermanence:

> *"Impermanence and change are thus the undeniable truths of our existence. What is real is the existing moment, the present that is a product of the past, or a result of the previous causes and actions. Because of ignorance, an ordinary mind conceives them all to be part of one continuous reality. But in truth they are not."*[78]

On paper, impermanence stands a solid argument, however, in practice, we either retire to a remote mountain, or we face the fact that fantasising about a positive abundant future is a great exercise to address potential fear. In addition, discovering that, instead of addressing my fear, I was just pushing against it with a now-or-never mentality, I was negating myself to dream big.

Why are we afraid to have it all?

To put ourselves first?

To say 'no'?

I am not saying that letting my imagination loose will manifest Ryan Reynolds at my door (that said, I would not mind that at all). What I am saying is that by believing that we can have it all, and remembering there is *nothing* wrong in wanting it all does not mean that I am greedy or against mindful living. Instead, it's a way to celebrate our hard work by reminding ourselves that we are reaping the benefits of our daily hustle.

Living in the now shall not preclude you from accepting you are meant to be, do, have great things. Saying yes to incredible opportunities should not prevent you from saying 'no' when something does not feel right.

Sabotage Alert: Should you say No more often? With Hannah Rose Cluley

My bestie has this question she loves to ask, "Is it a hell yes? Because if it's not a hell yes, then it's a hell no".

Let's look at that word, No.

It's such a powerful word, and you'd also like to know that the books written about the importance of saying 'yes' or 'no' (depending on the argument of the author, obviously) is higher than what you'd ever expect.

Our life is shaped by questions, as we discussed in Habit One. As much as asking questions we also make countless decisions each day. From which kind of milk we should buy, to what to do about a business meeting, we must learn to say no to the things that do not serve us so that we can say yes to the things that truly light us up.

Now, you may be reading this, my Dear Reader, and thinking that it all sounds quite on point, however, saying no to things gets harder and harder, the more our online influence grows.

It's just common sense: the more we are present online, sharing our message and our skillsets, the more people would want to be part of that vision.

However, I want you to see your No's as a true act of love towards yourself. By saying No, you tap into that feeling of inner abundance. You know you are/have/do enough, and you do not have to take on something new but you want to do it. It's the basic ability of perceiving the abundance in your life and being compassionate towards yourself by allowing yourself to rest.

Do not say yes as a way to fill your time and space with noise. The utter fear of being bored is something that can prevent us from growth. Seriously, when is the last time you sat in silence, doing nothing? If you can't remember, it's been too long.

I do not even mean meditating. I mean simply enjoying nothingness. Being bored is a feeling my generation still was familiar with - I am finding that now it would be actually very hard to feel bored, as it would require is to actively seek boredom. Maybe that is what we are meant to do?

Be content with who we are and what we have, and making it our mission to be of service for others, using our influence for the - so called - greater good.

At the end of the day you decide whether to see your glass half full of kombucha, or half empty - I am so sorry, I could not resist.

I caught up with the gorgeous Hannah Rose Cluley (@hannahrosecluley) to discuss everything kindness and vulnerability. Yoga teacher, self-lover and influencer, Hannah is also one of the funniest people I know - what can I say, I tend to surround myself with pretty hilarious people.

I asked her about saying no and being vulnerable online.

When do you think saying NO is important for your own wellbeing?

I think as a freelancer, you're constantly being driven to book jobs. To shake hands. To keep a stream of things coming in. The freedom we get from working for ourselves also brings uncertainty, and I know for myself and many other people I've spoken to who also work for themselves, the fear of not getting enough work is a big thing. So we say yes, a lot. Especially when we're new to the freelance world.

Being your own boss, and having to be proactive about getting an income is actually pretty stressful, and I truly believe that freelancers have it tough. We work a lot harder than many people who are employed, because we do the work, we also get the clients and we have to manage everything behind the scenes. This is also great and is why many people love the working for yourself life, but it can be problematic. If you're a 'yes' person like me, you say yes to pretty much everything.

Yes is a great word, it opens you up to so many awesome opportunities, but No is just as, if not more important, because the No is what will really save you as a freelancer. Learning to say No is vital, the No will protect your physical health, it will protect your mental health, it will protect your social health (relationships with others), and it will protect your work and your brand. Because by saying No, and not taking on too much, you're not compromising the quality of what you produce, you're not affecting how you come across as a business, and you're not going to be overworking and causing damage to your body and mental wellbeing.

How do you think social media has allowed us to be more vulnerable?

Social media is an amazing place, particularly when it comes to getting vulnerable and digging deep. For me, social media is almost like a journal, I use it to write out how I feel and it's very cathartic. We as humans tend to find it hard to get vulnerable, our inner ego is always trying to protect itself, and opening up to those we're close to in life can seem really bloody scary.

I personally think that the more followers you have, the easier it gets. In our minds, the moment the number starts to hit 10,000+, when Instagram stops showing your following as a 4 digit number, but as two (or three with a decimal point) digits with a 'K', is the moment your followers seem less like actual real humans. And I don't mean that in a bad way, I mean, it's much easier to open up to a number, through a virtual online platform, where you can sit in your living room and write about the rubbish day you've had, than it would be to sit across from a friend and really bare your soul, emotions raw and ready to be seen by another real life human being.

Social media also puts us onto a platform, think theatre stage, lights are shining on you, and the audience is in total darkness. The anonymity of the audience definitely helps.

As well as all of this, when we start to get vulnerable (and most of us start small at first), we start to get feedback from those followers. Usually the feedback is "you've helped me so much, I feel the same" or "it's so good to know that I'm not alone here". This feedback acts as positive reinforcement and encouragement, and gradually we continue to open up and dig deeper.

These different variables are things that aren't usually present away from social media, which is what makes it such a special and significant thing in terms of vulnerability.

What is the downside, if any, of openness and vulnerability online, on platforms full of hundreds of strangers?

The downside of getting vulnerable in this way, is that first of all, we start to almost feel a responsibility. This positive feedback and reinforcement is great, but it also shows us that people really do appreciate the words we say, and we start to feel like they almost rely a little bit on that. This coupled up with the fact that it is a release and it is cathartic for us, means that we probably share much more with people than we ordinary would in such a public setting. We don't keep anything to ourselves, unless we set strict boundaries, which can be hard, coming from someone who really enjoys sharing and opening up.

Energy isn't just something that's present in a room, it can be transmitted through social media, and it is totally possible to give too much energy out, without being able to replenish your own cup.

When should we ask for help, and when does our community help with that?

The time to ask for help is the moment you realise things are too much. Reach out to friends, text someone, call your mum, write to a FB group you're part of. Vulnerability isn't just cathartic, vulnerability and opening up about when things have gone too far, will literally save you.

There are so many groups on Facebook and communities like the Health Bloggers Community where you can meet and talk to like-minded people who are going through the same thing.

Why do you think we struggle with asking for help?

We're human, and therefore being vulnerable is hard. Asking for help is just another facet of vulnerability, which isn't an easy thing to do. We always want to protect ourselves as best we can, and showing that we are struggling can often feel too raw and too real, so by not reaching out, we are able to pretend everything is fine.

PART THREE: ACTION STEPS + CONCLUSION

The 21-Day
Action Plan

As I mentioned *endless* times, "repetition is the mother of skills". Moreover, pretty words on paper do not magically translate into action. Actions themselves propel miracles to happen. This is why all I am asking you to do is to use this action plan as a checklist. For the next four weeks do one of these things, one day at a time.

Give it a go. Get a fresh journal, your favourite pen and let me know your progress at @fabgiovanetti or by using the hashtag #makeanimpactbook

Prep Work: How to cultivate a habit

Before you start: Plant the seed and be disciplined

Before getting started with your action steps, take time to dissect your habits. What is your trigger? What routine do you want to change or develop, and what will be your reward?

In order to cultivate habits you must be able to understand how to implement it and get your reward - it comes down to practise, self-awareness as well as clear ways to measure your improvements. Grab your journal and write down what you are looking to get out of these 4 weeks. Be specific, have a clear goal to measure again, make sure it's relevant and has a clear deadline to keep you accountable.

Day one: How to find your Why

Before even getting started with your goals and tasks, it's time to get back to your why. Consciously invest time in getting back to your Why and you'll find yourself less frazzled, demotivated and scattered.

Below there are my three favourite questions to define your why:

- What is your mission?

- How do you want to help others?

- For what do you want to be remembered?

5-Minute Action Step: Answer these questions in your journal and refine your why. Make it bold, grandiose and sparkling - feel free to use some glitter in there as well. After you write your why down, make sure you have it somewhere very clear that you can see it in every day (your vision board, mirror or desk will do).

Day Two: The Golden Circle

Once you have a clear Why, it's time to give it some context. The best exercise to give yourself some sense of direction comes from *Start with Why* by Simon Sinek, and it's linked to a very special Circle - a Golden one. The Golden Circle consists of three concentric circles with the *Why* being the main yolk, the *How* wrapped around that like an egg white, and the *What* as the outermost circle.

5-Minute Action Step: Create your Golden Circle starting from your why.

Day Three: Setting Clear Goals

I always recommend setting one big goal, and a daily, small actionable goal you'll achieve before anything else.

Ask yourself: what am I going to achieve today to get one step closer to my Why?

Write down the whole list, then start prioritising. I am not here to tell you how to write your daily tasks, mainly as I am aware it differs from person to person. Just make sure your main action step is at the top, and that that one task is what you are going to prioritise for the day.

5-Minute Action Step: Write down the one task you'll get done first thing tomorrow, and give it your complete attention.

Day Four: Set a Power Hour

Let's be honest here, we all have the innate ability avoid the most important thing YOU needed to work on. It does not matter if it is a phone call or a project for a client, for yourself, or just something that needed to get done. You do everything BUT what you are meant to do. It's just the way we feel we are "being "productive. By crossing things off a list instead of doing the important stuff first.

The most incredible thing about this hour (the Power Hour you all), is that it sounds much easier than it is. In that hour, you will not let distractions such as unnecessary breaks, kettle rounds, emails, social media, or INSTAGRAM suck you in the procrastination spiral.

5-Minute Action Step: Take your main goal for the day, and focus your whole Power Hour on it, and see how your productivity changes.

Day Five: Practise Storytelling

To craft a great story you need context, action and the result (CAR). And what's true for academics is as true for influencers. A lot of people can get hung up on the context. When you're establishing context, it's important that you try your best to ensure that your audience can relate to your story as much as possible.

This means that, if telling a story, make sure you have a clear point you are trying to put across. All you have to do, it create a good mixture of success and failure, as well as aiming to give back to your audience by providing them with something tangible they can action themselves through the conclusion to your story.

I love networking events for this sort of exercise.

5-Minute Action Step: Find an event that looks enticing enough, and go there on your own. After introducing yourself to other people in the room, practice telling people about your mission and how you are planning to make an impact. The more you practice your story, asking others questions about themselves, and incorporating direct experience, the better you will become at influencing others.

Day Six: Asking the Right Questions

Today is the day you tackle a problem, issue, worry that has been on your mind for a while and you have been procrastinating on. A lot of the times, the most important tool you have are questions. Once you know the questions, HOW you answer can be easily improved by learning how to tell a story that can facilitate your answer.

I am listing a few questions I always find extremely valuable, especially in moments of hardship:

4. What can I do today to get from A to B?

5. What have we not tried yet, to solve this problem?

6. What are all the benefits you'll gain by taking action?

7. How will this decision enhance your life?

5-Minute Action Step: Write down a pressing problem you have been trying to solve. Take time to ask yourself any of these questions that you think may help you solving this problem.

Day Seven: You are your Main Product

You don't have to be your own brand: you can see the coaches, the nutritionists and the personal trainers choose their name as a way to create some legacy that can be translated into speaking opportunities, books and other opportunities.

Stand for something bigger: more and more influencers are launching their own campaign or brand alongside their own mission, as a way to create an extra degree of separation, and also harness the power of community and collaboration. This can really help you reiterating your mission, as well as go beyond yourself in order to create a tighter relationship with your audience.

5-Minute Action Step: Who do you want to be? Whichever avenue you decide to pursue, take the next five minutes to decide how you want people to perceive your brand.

Day Eight: Moving on From Failure

Keep track of your projects, and assess their overall performance. If something is not working anymore, ask yourself what has changed and assess whether it's time to adapt or let it go:

- Once you decide what to let go of, give yourself some time to have a little wiggle, a cry or a tub of ice-cream (or even having a friend on call) and accept that it's time to move on.

- What have you learnt from this experience: what will you repeat, and what should you not do again?

- What's next for you? Write down what is your current focus, and where you'll put your energies in.

5-Minute Action Step: Ask yourself, is there anything I can let go of right now? Find that thing and go through the 3-step process.

Day Nine: Diversify your Content

I would always recommend build two to three media minimum, one of which must be your own (aka your website or email list). Others can be Instagram, YouTube, and Twitter etc. All of those who own everything you do, post or share. If you are not ready to sell yet, this is a way you can start diversifying from the get-go.

Content-avenues:

- Newsletter
- Website
- Blog
- Podcast
- YouTube
- Instagram
- Twitter
- Facebook

5-Minute Action Step: Write down in your journal 2/3 content avenues. How often will you post there? What type of content will people expect to see? Write three options for each avenue, and start building your calendar from it.

Day Ten: Diversify your Income

Do not be fooled: just because something worked for a number of years, it does not mean it will always do. Instead of breaking down every single service, I like to diversify income-avenues as follows:

- Seasonal Income
- Time-bound project
- Recurring Active Income
- Passive Income
- Recurring Passive Income
- One-off Fee

Now, because I feel I went deep down the rabbit hole of the business side of things, let me provide you with some examples for each one of those:

- Seasonal Income
- Events
- Time-bound project
- Sponsored Post
- Recurring Active Income
- Management / Monthly Content Creation
- Passive Income
- eBook

- Recurring Passive Income
- Membership
- One-off Fee
- Speaking Fee

5-Minute Action Step: Even if you do not have loads of services / different income streams just yet, take the time to envision 2 or 3 different options you'd like to develop, and how they'll work together in a cohesive and balanced way.

Day Eleven: Should I start this New Project?

This is the day where I want you to think about a new opportunity, possibility or project that may have come your way recently. I want you to brainstorm how to assess whether this new opportunity is relevant to your Why, your mission and your goals.

Questions to ask yourself before taking on a new project:

1. Is it in line with my overall mission and why?

2. Does it feel like a 'hell yeah'?

3. Is it going to support / help my audience?

4. What's the commitment involved?

If it ticks all the boxes, you are good to go.

5-Minute Action Step: Write down the new opportunity and take five minutes to answer the four questions. I would say, if it does not feel like a "hell yeah", most times you do not need to explore the possibility further.

Day Twelve: Credibility and Breaking Trust

Let's talk about making mistakes - my best advice is always the same, regardless: be honest, be transparent, and let people know what's going on. Rather than frantically trying to fix the matter as soon as possible, give people a heads up, and take your time in order to ensure you know what happened and what you are looking to fix.

Here's why, my plan of action to deal with issues / complaints / comment is always the same.

1. Keep it private whenever possible - think private messages or emails.

2. Make sure you have a good argument to back up your opinions, whenever you are sharing some

3. Have a clear complaint 'contingency plan' that allows you to share your view-point with your audience.

5-Minute Action Step: What's your contingency plan? Make sure you have written down a clear plan of action for you to make sure you can handle any question coming your way. Better safe than sorry, I like to say.

Day Thirteen: Develop Expertise

Despite the fact that degrees and PhDs are an incredible asset and should be always considered, I believe there are so many ways to keep on developing your expertise:

- You can follow yourself people with great influence and expertise

- You can listen to podcasts and watch TED talks

- You can read books, attend seminars and read studies

- You can write essays, studies and research

- You can embark a new journey with a new degree, course or study path

- You can network, head to a conference or a workshop

5-Minute Action Step: today pick one thing you can do to work on your expertise and put it in your calendar.

Day Fourteen: Create Credible Content

Content and the way content is presented are as important as your footnotes, especially as you do not want to alienate people who are coming to you with a problem to solve, or an issue to resolve. I call this the "triple-whammy of credible influencers" (I know, I do have a talent for catchy names):

- trustworthiness (how believable the content is)
- clarity (how easily the content can be understood)
- accuracy (how well documented the content is)

Challenge yourself by thinking about people you can tap into that can support you in areas you do not know, and find reliable resources for your articles and posts.

5-Minute Action Step: Create a list of blogs, publications and websites to consult when discussing a very specific topic you want to support with further reading.

Day Fifteen: Facilitate Community Interaction

What are the building blocks of a community, the ones that you should have in order to nurture your very own?

- A leader (that's you, that is)

- A strong message to share

- A group of people to share this message to

There are so many other ways you can facilitate community interaction - here's a few examples, just to put things into perceptive:

- Twitter chats

- Instagram Live

- Webinar

- Facebook Live

- Collaborative Articles

- Interviews

- Speaking at an Event

5-Minute Action Step: announce your first Q&A or live and make sure you put the date in your calendar. This is a simple way to get people to know you.

Day Sixteen: How to Learn Something New

We all know by now that learning comes in many forms, and should be approached as a way to keep up with what is happening around you.

- Practise

- Motivation

- Mentors

Ways you can invest in yourself and your learning:

- Attend a seminar / workshop

- Join a book club

- Listen to audio books

- Listen to podcasts

- Have a list of monthly books you want to read

- Join a mastermind

- Curate an RSS feed with your favourite publications

5-Minute Action Step: today write down a list of 3 books that you've been meaning to read that you know can help you with your development and learning.

Day Seventeen: Find the Right Mentors

How do you go about finding a mentor?

The best thing is, nine times out of ten, to ask people out for a coffee.

If you are looking for a coach or a mentoring figure that can provide you with accountability, I recommend going to friends and peers in the community and ask for recommendations.

Another way to find mentors is to look at your current teachers and tutors, and ask them for some personal feedback or advice.

5-Minute Action Step: invite someone out for a coffee today - yes, it's that simple! Send someone you admire a DM or an email and get the conversation going.

Day Eighteen: Reassess your Core Values

Today is a day for us to reflect on things. I recommend everyone to revise their core values at least every six months. Values can be family, love, commitment, freedom, success, expansion and so on. Learning can often be mistaken as the need to learn something new about the world, when most often the best learning we can do is the one about ourselves.

5-Minute Action Step: what are core values after all? What are the three things that make your life better? Is if family, service, travel or love. At any given time we all have some specific values that shape our work and what we do.

Day Nineteen: Create Better Boundaries

When life throws you a curve ball or two, you got to breathe deeply and move on. The main action you can take is setting better and stronger boundaries - here's a few ideas on how to do so:

- Set an autoresponder with clear email times or turnaround time

- Add clear working hours to any agreement you send

- Do not check your email before/after a certain time

- Take notifications off your phone

- Delete social / email apps that you cannot stop checking

5-Minute Action Step: take your pick! Choose between one of the options above and start reclaiming your time in a more balanced way.

Day Twenty: Develop a Mindfulness practice

You know this was going to come up at some point - being able to cultivate self-awareness through a mindfulness practise is so important in order to be able to assess where you are at, what problems you are facing, and what you need to change.

5-Minute Action Step: whether you are potting a plant, journal for 5 minutes or do your first meditation session, make sure you embrace mindfulness in a new exciting way today.

Day Twenty One: Shake your Booty

Well, look at you! You are all done and dusted - I am so impressed. Today is my favourite day, today we dance. You may have heard rumours about my dancing skills (and these rumours are all true). I have loads of songs I love, but my manifesting song is called *Brave*. I love to sing it and dance my heart out.

5-Minute Action Step: get that music on and dance. Music is such an integral part of my life, I could not see my life without it. Today you are allowed to take your booty and celebrate your hard work.

This is the End

"Derek says it's always good to end a paper with a quote. He says someone else has already said it best. So if you can't top it, steal from them and go out strong. So I picked a guy I thought you'd like. 'We are not enemies, but friends. We must not be enemies. Though passion may have strained, it must not break our bonds of affection. The mystic chords of memory will swell when again touched, as surely they will be, by the better angels of our nature."

—DANNY VINYARD, AMERICAN HISTORY X

Finishing like I started: breaking that damn fourth wall.

If you could do only one thing for me today, let that be this. Lend this book to a friend who needs it - even better, *persuade* them to buy a copy of their own - wink.

Jokes aside, I really want this message to grow bigger and bigger, wider and wider. I want people with a big, bold message to feel less alone. I also want this conclusion to be different from a long stream of "thank-you"s - which, by the way, will be coming by the end of it, do not worry.

But this is not the end, oh no.

I want this to be the beginning. The beginning of what, you may ask? The beginning of one of those life-long friendships that are so improbable they were bound to happen - you know the ones I'm talking about, right?

People call me *mama Fab* for a reason. It's because I deeply care about people. It's because I want you, Dear Reader, my wonderful companion, to wake up in the morning and feel like you have a wonderful purpose and the drive to achieve whatever your heart desires.

I want you to know that nobody has it ever fully figured out, and that is okay.

I want you to remember that you are here for a reason, and you have one bloody shot at this, so you better make it a good one.

I want you to know that you are loved by many, and you sure enough are loved by me.

Because you are fricking awesome. Kick-ass. You have an incredible gift of making a positive impact, and I want you to never forget it.

Take it from the fiery but mighty Italian lady who had big dreams, loads of hopes, and no clue of how to get there.

Acknowledgements

I would not be here today without the support of my mum and my brother, all the family I have left, as well as my grandad, who I know is always here with me, and my dad, who allowed me to get out there in the world and do my thing, and somehow set me free.

Also wanted to thank my friends, in particular my bestie Hannah Wallace for believing in me, as well as introducing me to my publishers at That Guy's House - as well as Sean himself, for being an incredible beam of light, positivity and endless support from day one.

A very special sweaty hug goes to Samantha Couzens, without whom the HBC would not be still standing and thriving today: our laughs, your positive outlook and patience make me incredibly thrilled to go to work every day.

Of course, I also need to acknowledge and send buckets of love to my incredible backers: Flavia Croce, Rachel Bednarski, Emma Ahern, Hazel Wallace, Rebecca Pearson, Prabh Simran Badal, Ally Guppy, Kinga Perjes, , Luciana, Sarah Josefsberg, Rachel Evans, Camilla Dempster, Alexa R. Abraham, Eleonora Berra, Moriam Mustapha, Lisa-Jane Holmes, Lisa Targett, Delicia Bale, Amie Dawson, Fifi Mills, Laura Rua, Katharine Carter,

Donna Crous, Magdalena Pytlas, Sarah Orecchia, Kim Ingleby, Stephanie Perritone, Natascia Bernardi, Rachel Mar, Gessica Bicego, the ladies behind Naughty Nutrition, Susan Thirakornratch, Jessica Johansen, Jo Hodson, Katerina Vasilaki, Lashara van Heerden, Ceri Jones, Paula Heaney, Joanna Konstantopoulou.

Bibliography

1000 True Fans, Online, Kelly, Kevin. https://kk.org/thetechnium/1000-true-fans/

12 Rules for Life: An Antidote to Chaos, Peterson, Jordan B, Dr (2018)

7 Habits of Highly Effective People, Covey, Stephen (1989)

A More Beautiful Question: The Power of Inquiry to Spark Breakthrough Ideas, Berger, Warren (2014)

Contagious: Why things Catch On, Berger, Jonah (2013)

Daily Rituals: How Artists Work, Currey, Mason (2013)

Descriptive Social Norms and Motivation to Vote: Everybody's Voting and So Should You, Journal of Politics 71, 1–14; Frey, Bruno, and Stephan Meier (2004)

Digital media and youth:Unparalleled opportunity and unprecedented responsibility, In M. Metzger, & A. Flanagin (Editors), Digital media, youth, and credibility (pp. 5–28). Cambridge, MA: The MIT Press.

Feeling and form in groups. Visual Sociology, Sandelands, L. E. (1998)

First Things First, Covey, Stephen R. Merrill, Roger. Merrill, Rebecca (1996)

Give Your Ideas Some Legs: The Positive Effect of Walking on Creative Thinking, Oppezzo, Marily. Schwartz, Daniel L. (2013)

Highly influential People and Influencers Survey, Fab Giovanetti (2017)

How Do People Adhere to Goals When Willpower Is Low? The Profits (and Pitfalls) of Strong Habits, Neal et al. (2013)

Influencer Marketing Report, Q1, Health Bloggers Community

Invisible Influence: The hidden forces that shape behaviour, Berger, Jonah (2016)

Lead with a Story: A Guide to Crafting Business Narratives that Captivate, Convince and Inspire, Smith, Paul (2012)

Leading Collaborations in Online Communities, Samer Faraj, Srinivas Kudaravalli , Molly Wasko, La Puma J, Marx RM. ChefMD's Big Book of Culinary Medicine. New York: Crown;

Making Habits, Breaking Habits: Why We Do Things, Why We Don't, and How to Make Any Change Stick, Dean, Jeremy (2013)

Motivational Interviewing: Helping People Change, 3rd Edition, William R. Miller and Stephen Rollnick (2013)

Neural Correlates of Lyrical Improvisation: An fMRI Study of Freestyle Rap https://www.nature.com/articles/srep00834

Oxford Handbook of Human Action, E. Morsella, J. A. Bargh, P. M. Gollwitzer, eds.,(New York: Oxford University Press, 2008).

Peer Effects with Random Assignment: Results for Dartmouth Roommates, Quarterly Journal of Economics 116, 681–704; Lerner, Josh, and Ulrike Malmendier (2013),

Purple Cow: Transform your Business by Being Remarkable, Godin, Seth (2003)

Singletasking: Get More Done - One Thing at a Time, Devora, Zack (2015)

Skill in chess, American Scientist, Volume 61 Number 4, Herbert Simon and William Chase, pp. 394-403 (1973)

Social Learning and Health Plan Choice, Sorensen, Alan T. RAND Journal of Economics 37, 929–45; Sacerdote, Bruce (2001)

Statistic Brain Institute, 2013 Attention Span Research, https://www.statisticbrain.com/

The Airbnb Story: How Three Ordinary Guys Disrupted an Industry, Made Billions . . . and Created Plenty of Controversy, Gallagher, Leigh (2017)

The Art of Influencing Anyone: Make People Do Whatever You Want, Cassidy, Niall (2013)

The Creators Code: The Six Essential Skills of Extraordinary Entrepreneurs, Wilkinson, Amy (2016)

The Death of Expertise, Nichols, Tom (2017)

The Ethics of Affective Leadership: Organizing Good Encounters Without Leaders, (p.53), Cambridge Quarterly, I Munro, T Thanem (2018)

The Four Horsemen of Automaticity: Awareness, Intention, Efficiency, and Control in Social Cognition. John A. Bargh, Handbook of Social Cognition, vol. 1: Basic Processes; vol. 2: Applications (2nd Ed.) Eds. R. S. Wyer and T. K. Srull (Hillsdale, NJ: Lawrence Erlbaum Associates, Inc., 1994), 1–40. (2006)

The Midnight Disease: The Drive to Write, Writer's Block, and the Creative Brain, Flaherty, Alice Weaver (2004)

The One Thing, Keller, Gary (2013)

The Power of Habit, Duhigg, Charles (2012)

The Story Factor, Simmons, Annette (2006)

The Tipping Point: How Little Things Can Make a Big Difference, Gladwell, Malcom (2002)

Tribes: We Need You to Lead Us, Godin, Seth (2008)

Trusting what you are told: How Children Learn from Others, Harris, Paul (2015)

The Ideal Team Player: How to Recognize and Cultivate the Three Essential Virtues, P Lencioni, Patrick (2016)

Wellspoken Research, Sarah Greenidge, 2017 Study

When being distracted is a Good Thing, Brogan, Jan (2012), https://www.bostonglobe.com/lifestyle/health-wellness/2012/02/27/when-being-distracted-good-thing/1AYWPlDplqluMEPrWHe5sL/story.html

Who, Smart, Geoff. Street, Randy (2008)

Wired for Stories, Cron, Lisa (2012)

Young Children Prefer and Remember Satisfying Explanations, Frazier, Brandy N. (2016)

Endnotes

[1]   Podcast, Tim Ferris Show, February 3rd, The Four Hour Work Week Revisited

[2]   Berger, Jonah. Invisible Influence: The hidden forces that shape behaviour (p. 60)

[3]   Authority Or Community? A Relational Models Theory Of Group-level Leadership Emergence P.596

[4]   Statistic Brain Institute, 2013 Attention Span Research

[5]   Berger, Jonah. Invisible Influence: The hidden forces that shape behaviour (pp. 88, 94)

[6]   Berger, Jonah. Invisible Influence: The hidden forces that shape behaviour (p. 15)

[7]   Berger, Jonah. Invisible Influence: The hidden forces that shape behaviour (p. 153)

[8]   Motivational Interviewing: Helping People Change, 3rd Edition, William R. Miller and Stephen Rollnick, 2013

[9]   Sandelands, L. E. Feeling and form in groups. Visual Sociology, 13: pp. 5–23.

[10]   Sandelands, L. E. 1998. Feeling and form in groups. Visual Sociology, 13: pp. 5–23.

11   Berger, Jonah. Invisible Influence: The hidden forces that shape behaviour (p. 2).

12   Gladwell, Malcolm. The Tipping Point (p. 21)

13   Berger, Jonah. Invisible Influence: The hidden forces that shape behaviour (p. 4)

14   Cambridge Dictionary, Online 2018

15   Berger, Jonah. Contagious, p.64

16   The Ethics of Affective Leadership: Organizing Good Encounters Without Leaders, p.53

17   https://www.psychologicalscience.org/news/were-only-human/ink-on-paper-some-notes-on-note-taking.html

18   E. Morsella, J. A. Bargh, P. M. Gollwitzer, eds., Oxford Handbook of Human Action

19   Buhigg , Charles .The Power of Habit (p.30)

20   Neal et al., (2013) How Do People Adhere to Goals When Willpower Is Low? The Profits (and Pitfalls) of Strong Habits

21   Eyal, Nir. Hooked: How to Build Habit-Forming Products (p. 1).

22   Buhigg , Charles .The Power of Habit (p.23)

23   Buhigg, Charles. The Power of Habit (p.48)

24   Cron, Lisa. Wired for Stories

25   Cron, Lisa. Wired for Stories

26   Smith, Paul. Lead with a Story

27   Cron, Lisa. Wired for Stories

28   YouTube, April 2018

29   Kurt Vonnegut, Letters http://www.worldcat.org/title/kurt-vonnegut-letters/oclc/775897860&referer=brief_results

30   Currey, Mason. Daily Rituals

31   Harris, Paul. Trusting What you are Told

32   Frazier, Brandy N. Young Children Prefer and Remember Satisfying Explanations

33   Sinek, Simon. Ted Talk "How Great Leaders Inspire Action"

34   EurekaAlert.org, New UTSA study describes how dopamin tells you it isn't worth th wait

35   Devora, Zack. Singletasking: Get More Done - One Thing at a Time

36   Cron, Lisa. Wired for Story (p.30)

37   The Balance Blonde Blog

38   Keller, Gary. The One Thing

39   Cambridge Dictionary, 2018

40   Covey, Stephen. First Things First

41   Frankl, Viktor. Man's Search for Meaning

42   Influencer Marketing Report, Q1

43   How Seth Godin Manages His Life — Rules, Principles, and Obsessions

44   https://seths.blog/2009/04/first-ten-/

45   Wilkinson, Amy. The Creators Code

46   Cassidy, Niall.The Art of Influencing Anyone

47   Cassidy, Niall.The Art of Influencing Anyone

48   Giovanetti, Fab. High Performers Survey

49   Wellspoken, 2017 Study

50   Giovanetti, Fab. High Performers Survey

51   Flanagin and Metzger (2008), Digital media and youth: Unparalleled opportunity and unprecedented responsibility. In M. Metzger, & A. Flanagin (Editors), Digital media, youth, and credibility (pp. 5–28). Cambridge, MA: The MIT Press.

52   Cassidy, Niall.The Art of Influencing Anyone

53   Oxford Dictionary, Online, 2018

54   Nichols, Tom. The Death of Expertise

55   Godin, Seth. Tribes: We need you to lead us (p. 10). Little, Brown Book Group. Kindle Edition.

56   Kelly, Kevin. 1000 True Fans, Online

[57]   Godin, Seth. Tribes: We need you to lead us (p. 28). Little, Brown Book Group. Kindle Edition.

[58]   Sinek, Simon. Start with Why

[59]   https://www.theboxmag.com/crossfit-training/origins-of-crossfit-9629

[60]   Duhigg, Charles.The Power of Habit (p.40)

[61]   Lencioni, Patrick. The Ideal Team Player

[62]   Lencioni, Patrick. The Ideal Team Player

[63]   Godin, Seth. Tribes: We need you to lead us (p.73)

[64]   Giovanetti, Fab. High Performers Survey

[65]   Cross reference between the High Performers and Influencers Surveys

[66]   Leading Collaboration in Online Communities, Samer Faraj , Srinivas Kudaravalli , Molly Wask

[67]   La Puma J, Marx RM. ChefMD's Big Book of Culinary Medicine. New York: Crown; 2008

[68]   Coyle, Daniel. The Talent Code

[69]   Skill in chess, American Scientist, Volume 61 Number 4 pp. 394-403, Herbert Simon and William Chase

[70]   Coyle, Daniel. The Talent Code

[71]   Covey, Stephen. 7 Habits of Highly Effective People

[72]   Covey, Stephen. 7 Habits of Highly Effective People

73   https://www.nature.com/articles/srep00834

74   Flaherty, Alice Weaver. The Midnight Disease

75   https://www.bostonglobe.com/lifestyle/health-wellness/2012/02/27/when-being-distracted-good-thing/1AYWPlDplqluMEPrWHe5sL/story.html

76   Give Your Ideas Some Legs: The Positive Effect of Walking on Creative Thinking, Marily Oppezzo and Daniel L. Schwartz

77   Smart, Geoff. Street, Randy. Who

78   (Urbandharma.org)